Well-Being and the Elderly: An Holistic View

Edited by Geralyn Graf Magan and Evelyn L. Haught

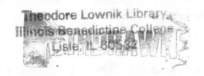

American Association of Homes for the Aging
1129 20th Street NW, Suite 400
Washington, DC 20036

The American Association of Homes for the Aging (AAHA), a national non-profit organization, represents nonprofit homes, housing, health-related facilities, and community services for the elderly. AAHA members are sponsored by religious, fraternal, labor, private, and governmental organizations committed to providing quality services for their residents and for elderly persons in the community at large.

The American Association of Homes for the Aging wishes to acknowledge the support of Summit Associated Marketing, Lee's Summit, Missouri, in the production of this book.

ISBN 0-943 774-27-6

Library of Congress Catalog Card No. 86-70934

Printed in the United States of America

The opinions expressed in this publication are solely those of the authors and do not reflect any official opinion of the American Association of Homes for the Aging.

Contents

Introduction

In his 1966 introduction to *The Social Components of Care* (Washington, D.C.: AAHA, 1966), the Rev. William T. Eggers, then vice president of the American Association of Homes for the Aging, referred to a macabre modern sculpture in describing the elderly and the care they receive in homes for the aging.

The sculpture depicted a man's body dotted with gaping holes. Just like the statue, Eggers observed, modern men and women are bombarded and invaded throughout their lives by external forces and pressures that gradually erode the total self. The bombardment continues through old age; for those entering homes for the aging, the traumatic transition from private to communal living—Eggers called it "the admission crisis"—often represents a culmination of those lifelong assaults on the individual.

The admission crisis is as real to the elderly person today as it was twenty years ago when Eggers recognized its potentially devastating effects. It involves a complex range of emotions, from anxiety to guilt, that are played out against the background of the imposing institution. That institution has the power either to make the invaded person whole again or to add to the assaults on him.

The institution's nature—its humanistic or religious stance, its understanding of the nature of man, its role as a social institution—concerned Eggers. He and other AAHA members like him felt strongly that the home for the aging had a responsibility to repair the worn spirit as well as to maintain the tired body. They turned those feelings into an approach to care—called the social components of care—which, to this day, forms the philosophical framework of the association.

The social components of care, as defined by Eggers, include those home arrangements—either physical or programmatic—that allow and encourage older people "fully to realize themselves both as individuals with personal dignity and as members of the home's community and of the larger community in which the home is located." Specifically, homes that offer the social components of care address the needs of the total person: social, emotional, psychological, spiritual, and physical.

This holistic philosophy represented a marked departure from the medical model of care—care of the body alone—practiced up to this time in many homes for the aging. While not devaluating the physical well-being of the elderly person, the social components of care suggest that other aspects of care—provision of a pleasant environment that respects human dignity, a social atmosphere devoid of myriad rules and regulations, and programs ad-

i

ministered by interdisciplinary teams of doctors, nurses, social workers, and clergy—can be combined to enhance the total well-being of the elderly person. The whole care program, then, is greater than the sum of its parts.

It seems appropriate that now, in its twenty-fifth year, the American Association of Homes for the Aging should reaffirm its commitment to the social components of care by publishing *Well-Being and the Elderly: An Holistic View*. While the term "holism"—the idea that integrated systems are more significant than the sum of their parts—may be new to AAHA's vocabulary, its meaning remains a comfortable one for the almost 3,000 homes and housing facilities that have offered the social components of care for many years. The holistic philosophy also describes AAHA's approach to community services.

In preparing this book, the American Association of Homes for the Aging sought to look in greater detail than ever before at care of the total person. The authors step beyond merely affirming the value of holistic care in order to suggest *practical* ways in which such care can be provided. In addition, the book expands upon the definition of the social components of care by recognizing that, in addition to advocating fulfillment of an individual's physical, psychological, social, and spiritual needs, holistic care requires that each program or system of care be part of an integrated system with specific goals and concepts.

Gregg Warshaw, M.D., begins the book with an examination of the most obvious need displayed by the elderly: the need for health care. He warns that health care of the elderly cannot be viewed as the treatment of an unrelated collection of aches and pains that a person must expect with old age. Rather, writes Warshaw, medical care of the elderly must take into consideration the body's entire medical and social system, including the patient's attitude about his or her physical condition and the status of his or her social support system.

David O. Moberg, Ph.D., follows Warshaw's examination of health care needs with a look at the spiritual needs that often become accentuated in late life. Physical decline, loss of friends and family, discrimination, and inflation take their toll on the older person's psyche, writes Moberg; however, when all else is in decline, there still can be growth toward greater spiritual maturity that can lighten the burdens and brighten the paths of the aging. No organization genuinely concerned with providing holistic care will neglect its role in providing avenues for this important growth, since any comprehensive spiritual care program is likely to affect positively every other aspect of the older person's life.

Lorraine G. Hiatt, Ph.D., in her chapter on environmental design, suggests that holistic environments help shape an older person's self-image, can either improve the quality of life or become agents in the aging process, can help prevent disability, stimulate thinking, and reduce agitation. Designing those environments, writes Hiatt, requires that the home step back from popular lists of design facts in order to provide an integrated system of services, architecture, and design.

Herbert J. Weiss, M.D., Rose Dobrof, D.S.W., Ira C. Robbins, A.C.S.W., and Cheryl Riskin, M.Ed., outline several holistic approaches to care of the mentally impaired elderly that often are applicable to the well-being of the nonimpaired person as well.

Herbert J. Weiss, M.D., suggests that a more holistic approach to the diagnosis of apparent dementia—one that assesses function and capacity for adaptive living—might result in more successful treatment. One of the important losses in old age, he maintains, is loss of the capacity to adapt physically to the environment and psychologically to impaired physical function and failing social resources. When this adaptive capacity fails, deficits that were previously present but were held in check by the momentum of adaptive living—unsolved emotional conflict, for example—are brought back to the surface in the form of severe dementia. Relief of that emotional conflict often can ease the pressures of physical symptoms.

This emphasis on capabilities, rather than deterioration, marks the cultural arts program described by Cheryl Riskin, M.Ed. The program offered sessions in literature, theater, vocal music, visual arts, and dance, helping both impaired and nonimpaired persons overcome their deficits by concentrating on what they *could* do. Residents wrote poetry, performed plays, sang and listened to music, enjoyed art as participants and observers, and learned to dance while remaining seated. Through the arts, the impaired were able to become active participants in life, learning to be productive and to feel success.

Dr. Rose Dobrof's holistic approach to care of the mentally impaired involves the creation of a therapeutic environment that maximizes the older person's capabilities while protecting that person from physical or emotional assault. This approach, writes Dobrof, requires that all staff—including aides, porters, maids, social workers, nurses, doctors, and occupational therapists—forsake their traditional statuses and rights in order to work as a unified force in caring for the mentally impaired. Ideally, this caring team also should include families of the mentally impaired elderly. These family members require tremendous support to deal with the horrendous feelings that beset them, but they have an unmatched ability to show the mentally impaired person that he or she is not alone.

Ira C. Robbins, A.C.S.W., offers myriad examples to illustrate Dobrof's team approach in his description of the holistic program of care he administered at Beth Sholom Home in Richmond, Virginia. The program included Reality Orientation sessions led by trained housekeepers and secretaries, various programs that provided personal contact between staff and residents, and an integrated program that attempted to create a humanized, stimulus-enriched atmosphere through physical exercise, stimulation of the senses, social interaction with children and with other residents, a sense of achievement through crafts and repetitious tasks, involvement of family, and perceptual environmental cues.

Just as Gregg Warshaw suggests that caring for the elderly involves more than treating a collection of unrelated aches, Peter V. Rabins, M.D., maintains that medications cannot be prescribed in a vacuum. The physician must respect the body as an integrated system whose balance often is disturbed by drugs improperly prescribed. Rabins discusses the effects that drugs can have on behavior, mood, and cognition and underscores the importance of proper diagnosis in the determination of which drugs to prescribe.

Terry F. Crawford, D.D.S., concludes the book with discussion of the area of care most overlooked in—and yet vital to—care of the total person: care of the teeth and mouth. Given the effects that dental health has on both self-image and overall health of the individual, it would be difficult to provide holistic care without paying proper attention to the oral cavity, writes Crawford. Dental care of the elderly, he maintains, should be offered as part of a total program that includes education of both staff and patients about the importance of oral hygiene, the training of staff and nonimpaired residents in brushing and flossing, and dental treatment which includes periodic health screening and comprehensive and emergency dental care.

William Eggers concludes his 1966 introduction to *The Social Components of Care* by recalling the Hans Christian Andersen fairy tale about the old street lamp "which had done its work for many, many years, but which was now to be pensioned off." The lamp worried about being useless or discarded and rejoiced when it was rescued and used by the family of an old watchman.

"They love me for myself," the fairy tale lamp concluded. "They have cleaned me and bought my oil. I am . . . well off now . . ." From that time, the lamp enjoyed more inward peace. And, the tale concludes, "the honest old Street Lamp had well deserved to enjoy it."

Like the watchman, nonprofit homes, housing, and community services can help the elderly find meaning, dignity, and love amid the terrible frustrations of aging. By respecting the older person as an individual, by recognizing the myriad needs that cry out to be met, by offering thoughtful care and services, we can pay tribute to those who well deserve to enjoy a productive and positive old age.

Chapter 1

Health Needs and the Elderly: Strategies for Effective Care

Gregg Warshaw, M.D.

The more we know about the problems of old age, the more exciting the potential contribution of modern medicine appears. Most important is the knowledge that many of the medical problems encountered by the elderly result not from the normal biological aging process but from controllable causes such as disease, a loss of ability resulting from inactivity, or the poverty and poor housing conditions that characterize the social position of many elderly people.

In general, elderly people are not dependent and disabled. To the contrary, the majority are active, self-reliant, and as independent as younger people. They are difficult to characterize because they represent a heterogeneous group, differing from one another in many more respects than they are similar. They differ also from the elderly of the past and future since the physical, psychological, and social conditions of older people change with each generation.

Today's elderly are, by and large, more fatalistic and pessimistic about their health than younger people. Many still believe that the problems that occur in old age are due to the aging process and that preventive measures and treatments are, therefore, unlikely to help.

The following review addresses the health needs of the elderly and strategies for providing effective care. Successful geriatric care should reach a variety of elderly patients: those who are healthy, those whose illness is unidentified, those who are acutely ill, and those who are chronically ill.

The Needs of Healthy Elderly People

Healthy elderly people have less need for medical investigation and treatment than they do for reassurance, information, and advice that will help them maintain and improve their health. Therefore, the most important contribution a health worker can make to an older person is to project good attitudes

Gregg Warshaw, M.D., is an associate professor, Geriatrics Division, in the Department of Family Medicine at the University of Cincinnati Medical Center and is also medical director of Maple Knoll Village in Springdale, Ohio.

about health promotion. The worker must be convinced that health and its pursuit are important, both to young and old. He or she must offer health advice that is practical, relevant, and likely to benefit the individual, based on the person's beliefs and attitudes. He or she must understand that the older person who asks, "What do you expect at my age?" may simply be echoing the health worker who once said, "What else do you expect at your age?"

Health Education

Health education should be tailored to the needs of each individual. However, the clinician should keep some useful general principles in mind:

- Before giving advice or information, listen to the older person's opinions about health. The older person's beliefs and attitudes are more influential than epidemiological evidence.
- Be brief. Long messages are easily forgotten.
- Keep it simple. One or two simple points may be remembered. Complex messages rarely are retained. Language should be fashioned so it can be understood by those with limited education.
- Be clear. Verbosity and jargon are useless.
- Be specific. Vague exhortations are less likely to be effective than specific prescriptions.
- Keep it relevant. Advice that does not relate to the individual circumstances is not likely to be followed.
- Reinforce the message. Repetition is important.

There are a number of relevant health education messages, some of which are listed below:

- Encourage increased consumption of fiber and calcium and decreased consumption of calories.
- Encourage elderly people to maintain and, if necessary, increase the amount of exercise taken to maintain and increase strength, skill, stamina, and suppleness.
- Encourage an annual visit to the dentist.
- Encourage visits for vision testing at least once every two years and sooner if vision fails.
- Encourage early consultation when hearing impairment becomes noticeable.
- Encourage the use of a qualified podiatrist or chiropodist if the person has circulatory problems or diabetes.

An important maxim always must accompany any health education message to an elderly person: "Old age is not a disease; it is never too late to improve your health."

2

Hidden Health Care Needs

Elderly persons can exhibit two types of hidden health needs.

The first are hidden from the patient. These asymptomatic diseases most often are detected through preventive strategies such as screening for hypertension or cancer.

The second group of needs is hidden from the doctor but not from the patient. These symptomatic diseases are undetected for a number of reasons. The elderly person may not think his or her medical problem is legitimate or remediable or may think such problems are to be expected with old age. Communication difficulties that stem from hearing or memory losses, or acute illness that can cause varying degress of confusion, may limit an older person's ability to seek help and to describe his or her problems clearly.

Health workers also can fail to detect problems because they, like the patient, attribute symptoms to aging. A physician examining a patient with hypothyroidism can be misled by its atypical presentation, a painless myocardial infarction or fracture can go undetected, or the physician can use a longstanding problem to explain a new pathology. For example, carcinoma of the colon may be overlooked if the symptoms are attributed to a patient's chronic constipation.

Prevention

Many of these hidden health problems can be detected through application of traditional preventive strategies. However, a better understanding of the scope of prevention as it applies to older people is fundamental to successful application of these strategies.

In the elderly, four groups of potentially preventable clinical problems can be identified:

1. Problems that can be addressed in traditional prevention terms, including diseases that fit into usual primary, secondary, and tertiary prevention categories. Such prevention would include screening for hypertension, cancer, or osteoporosis. Primary prevention stategies would include immunization for tetanus or influenza.

2. Behaviors likely to produce beneficial or adverse effects on health status. Risk-factor modification might include counseling on smoking, diet, and exercise.

3. Problems requiring attention from caregivers in the form of case finding. This would include the early identification and care of common clinical problems with vision, hearing, dentition, depression, dementia, alcoholism, and others.

4. Iatrogenic problems caused by medical care itself. Limiting iatrogenic problems may be the most promising area for prevention with the elderly.

3

Clinicians need to be alert to the risks of medication side effects and interactions and the potential complications of diagnostic or therapeutic interventions.

To progress toward a rational and effective preventive approach for geriatric care, clinicians must begin grappling with the complexities of applying anticipatory strategies to this age group. This application, aided by our expanded and improved ability to collect and organize useful data on elderly patients, forms the basis of "good" health care for the aged, which includes an emphasis on restoring function, avoiding iatrogenesis, and maintaining a community orientation.

Acute Health Care Needs

The treatment of acute disease is a major part of medical practice and training and consumes a high proportion of health care budgets.

In all age groups, the impact of an acute illness is determined by its nature and severity. In an older person it is additionally influenced by:
- the aging process itself, which causes a loss of reserve
- the loss of fitness that results from reduced mobility
- social and psychological features relating both to the individual and his or her environment
- the accessibility and utilization of health and social services.

Hospital Care

Many acute episodes are managed successfully by the elderly patient with or without the help of informal or formal services. However, some episodes inevitably lead to hospital admission. While many acutely ill elderly people actually need skilled in-patient medical care, others are admitted to a hospital because their social support systems have broken down.

The decision to admit an older person to the hospital often is necessary and justified. This is largely due to the fact that elderly patients admitted to the hospital with acute problems usually have a high prevalence of functional disability. Failure to admit to the hospital early enough might reduce the potential for this person's functional recovery. On the other hand, we must recognize that not many acute hospitals are designed or staffed to cope with the specific needs of the elderly. Hospitalization may have a negative impact on functional recovery even when the medical and surgical interventions are successful. In some cases, elderly patients who are precariously in touch with their surroundings are predisposed to confusion when they enter the hospital. The disorienting events of admission can accelerate this mental decline.

Geriatric Medicine

Geriatric medicine is an approach to general medical care of the elderly that is concerned with the clinical, preventive, remedial, and social aspects of illness in the elderly. It is not a discipline separate from the everyday practice of most clinicians; it requires only that caregivers keep in mind basic principles of good geriatric care while administering general medical care (D.C. Kennie. *JAMA* 1983: 770-773). Among these principles are the following:

- There is an increasing body of knowledge specific to the medical care of older patients.
- The success of care should be measured with an emphasis on restoration of function.
- Care and rehabilitation must allow sufficient time for healing and repair of older tissues.
- Older patients are increasingly at risk of side effects from diagnostic and therapeutic interventions; the prevention of iatrogenic illness is a constant concern for geriatricians.
- It is impossible to care adequately for older patients without being concerned about their social, family, financial, and psychological support systems.

Disease Presentation

When the elderly become sick, their clinical presentations often diverge from the classical accounts of disease. Presentations may be divided into several subgroups: absent, silent, atypical, and catastrophic.

Absent: Many old people simply do not complain about symptoms that would have brought a younger patient to the doctor earlier. An example of this "absent" presentation is painful knees, which may be attributed to "old age" by the patient but may actually be a remediable source of distress.

Silent: Older people have a diminished awareness of pain, which leads to the "silent" presentation. A painless heart attack is not unusual in an older patient; a nonspecific symptom such as poor appetite, nausea, or breathlessness may be its only manifestation.

Atypical: Ill elderly do not always show the symptoms commonly associated with their conditions. Hyperthyroidism in the elderly, for example, is often unaccompanied by an enlarged gland or eye changes. A rapid, irregular heartbeat or some confusion might be the only clue. Confusion also may be the most evident feature of hypothyroidism. Depression in an elderly patient may masquerade as dementia.

Catastrophic: Catastrophic presentation is the result of a general reduction in the elderly person's physical reserve and physiological function. This reduction makes the older individual prone to a dramatic, multisystem disease presentation. Falls, incontinence, and acute confusion frequently represent "catastrophic" presentations in previously well older people. These are nonspecific presentations of illness that require alert and careful evaluation. Proper assessment of these presentations depends upon a good patient history and the physician's awareness of the precarious nature of mobility, continence, and orientation in elderly patients. It is crucial to remember that good care often requires an urgent response on the part of the health worker.

After Hospital Discharge

Elderly patients recently discharged from the hospital can be forgotten or undersupervised since it is assumed that the acute problem has been resolved. In addition, when the primary health team is not formally involved with hospital care, its members may not be immediately aware of the discharge. Because relationships between hospital health workers and their community counterparts are frequently unclear, planning for the transfer of care often is deficient, particularly when the need to discharge a patient is urgent. Efforts should be made to:

- Ensure that all relevant members of the primary care team are aware of the discharge. One member of the team should visit the older person at home within a few days of discharge, particularly if the person's functional ability has significantly declined as a result of the disease that led to the admission. Functional ability and recovery can only be accurately addressed at home.
- Make certain that the person is taking the discharge medication in the manner prescribed. Mistakes in compliance commonly occur at this time. This is a good time to clear out the medicine cabinet to ensure that, in addition to medicine prescribed in the hospital, the patient does not resume the treatment he or she was receiving before hospital admission.

Chronic Health Care Needs

The main objectives of care for those with chronic health problems are:

- to help the individual maintain his or her quality of life
- to support relatives and other helpers
- to arrest or slow down the rate at which functional ability is lost.

The last objective is of particular importance. Questions such as, "Can you reach the toilet in time?" and "Can you get to the store?" are important in old age. Care, not cure, is the main objective when treating chronic illness. Effective rehabilitation may be the most effective preventive strategy available to the clinician.

Promoting Independence

An important concern in the provision of caring services for the elderly is maintaining a careful balance between promoting independence and creating dependency. Intervention and the addition of support too early are wasteful uses of limited resources and may, in themselves, diminish functional independence and intrude on the individual's privacy. On the other hand, delayed or inappropriate intervention can increase the prevalence of problems for the elderly person and lead to an avoidable hospital or institutional admission.

By educating home health workers and relatives not to do too much for elderly people, the clinician can help those elderly continue to make decisions and be active and continue to receive that important occupational therapy and physiotherapy that looking after themselves offers. There is too much "taking care of" elderly people when they have a right to struggle and a right to be at risk. The health worker often has to act as an advocate in defense of these rights.

The degree of a person's motivation is an extremely important factor in determining the potential for improving his or her functional ability. Not all elderly people are highly motivated to remain independent, and some may even refuse offers of treatment and rehabilitation. For some, this lack of motivation may reflect a lifelong personality trait; for others, it may represent a new characteristic. When an active and lively elderly person becomes apathetic and resigned, possible explanations for such a change—such as depression—should be investigated.

Death
Death, inevitably, becomes an issue for older individuals and their families. There is often an unstated desire for a "comfortable" death at home, free of the misplaced "heroics" that can occur with the inappropriate use of modern medical technology. Most of all, the vast majority of older individuals wants to remain as independent as possible. This means that health care resources should be used only when elderly persons want them and are likely to benefit from them.

Understanding Disease
For elderly patients and their relatives, diagnosis and treatment of chronic diseases may be less important than a full appreciation of what the problem means, how it will affect the individual, and how it is likely to progress. This understanding is particularly important in the early stages of dementia.

The routine assessment of patients with chronic problems requires a structured approach to ensure that no important issues are overlooked. Checklists and other assessment protocols should be used, particularly if they are cost-effective and feasible.

There are three main components to assessment:
- Establishing the diagnosis(es). This requires that the health worker appreciate the atypical clinical presentations seen in the elderly, the tenden-

cy of elderly persons to have multiple pathologies, the diseases that are specific to the elderly, and the importance of iatrogenic disorders.

- Evaluating the patient's functional status. This assessment should concentrate on the main activities of daily living, including mobility and walking, rising and transferring, continence, and dressing and feeding.
- Evaluating the patient's social support system.

When the decision has been made to admit an elderly patient to sheltered residential care or to a nursing home, the health team can facilitate the transition, which represents a major social upheaval for most old people. Every person in need of long-stay residential care should have a multidisciplinary assessment before admission. A physician should be involved whenever possible. He or she may detect treatable diseases responsible for the decline in functional ability that has led the older person to be labeled as "failing to cope" and in need of supervised care. Reassessment should take place routinely in the long-term care institution, since the state of health of an old person varies over time.

Rehabilitation

Rehabilitation can be broadly defined as an attempt by all health care personnel to encourage the patient to the fullest physical, mental, and social functioning. Such encouragement has been successful in enabling large numbers of patients of all ages to live independently in the community. Three groups of older patients requiring rehabilitation can be identified:

- those suffering from an obvious disorder, such as stroke or amputation, that affects functions
- those with a general systemic disorder such as severe cardiovascular or respiratory disease
- those who have no obvious disorder but who suffer from the accumulative effects of frailty in old age.

One of the essentials of rehabilitation is "progressive patient care," a system that classifies and separates patients according to their total health care needs. This is not only a more effective way to treat patients but also an efficient use of staff and resources.

In any setting or environment where rehabilitation takes place, such as long-term care settings, patients with multiple disorders and many different needs are grouped together. It becomes extremely difficult for the staff, no matter how well trained, to deal with any one disorder effectively. As an example, consider three elderly patients. One patient had a stroke two weeks ago, has minimal paralysis, and only needs assistance in dressing, putting on her leg brace, and going to the physical therapy department. Another patient is very confused and repeatedly tries to climb out of bed over the bed rail. A third is dying, is at risk of developing pressure sores, and has to be turned

8

every few hours. If faced with caring for all three patients, staff naturally will spend more time with the second and third patients, giving the patient requiring rehabilitation relatively little attention. In order to improve rehabilitation, patients with true rehabilitation potential should be concentrated in one area of the facility, allowing staff to work intensively with them.

Summary

This chapter has highlighted those areas of clinical practice that possess the potential for improving care of older patients.

We already know much about the clinical care of the elderly, what they need and want, and what works. We understand that effective care is the foundation of all clinical practice and, given the unique features of health problems in the elderly, health care can be both demanding and professionally challenging. Assessment and management of problems in older people require a high standard of clinical skills as well as an expanded view of health to include functional ability, fitness, socioeconomic status, and psychological functions. Learning those skills helps the clinician improve job satisfaction, increase motivation, and improve the care he or she provides on a daily basis.

Acknowledgments

This work was partly sponsored by the Kellogg International Program on Health and Aging, School of Social Work, The University of Michigan, and the Institute of Social Medicine, The University of Copenhagen.

Portions were adapted from: G. Almind, C. Freer, J.A. Muir Gray, and G. Warshaw, "The contribution of the primary care doctor to the medical care of the elderly in the community," *Danish Medical Bulletin* 32, Supplement Number 2 (1985): 1-32.

Chapter 2

Spirituality, Aging, and Spiritual Care

David O. Moberg, Ph.D.

"Care for the whole person," "total wellness," "holistic health services," and similar phrases have become popular slogans in human service programs and agencies. The philosophy of the American Association of Homes for the Aging rightly recognizes that this emphasis upon quality of life involves meeting older persons' physical, social, psychological, emotional, and spiritual needs, aiming "to help make life more meaningful for the aging." Yet, it is easy to overlook aspects of human need like spirituality because they are relatively intangible, have not been covered in professional education, seem to fall outside the domain of normal staffing patterns, and are not covered by conventional reimbursement sources.

In all too many agencies and programs for the aging, there is little direct concern for meeting spiritual needs, despite the fact that they comprise the most significant area of life in which continuing development is possible in the later years. When all else is in decline, there still can be growth toward greater spiritual maturity; this growth can lighten the burdens and brighten the paths of the aging while making the work of their caregivers easier and more rewarding.

Following a discussion of the nature and scope of spirituality, we shall briefly summarize data on the religiosity of the aging, spiritual needs in late life, the neglect of spiritual care, and research on spirituality. Then we shall suggest some guidelines and precautions that apply to spiritual care services.

The Nature and Scope of Spirituality

It is impossible through scientific methodologies to prove that human beings are spiritual creatures, for the spirit cannot be directly observed with the human senses. It must be remembered, however, that numerous other phenomena that are empirically unobservable have become the subjects of scientific investigation. These include space, time, alienation, depression, empathy, intelligence, loneliness, and pain, to mention but a few examples. The

David O. Moberg, Ph.D., is professor of sociology at Marquette University, Milwaukee, Wisconsin. He is the author of the Spiritual Well-Being *background paper for the 1971 White House Conference on Aging,* Wholistic Christianity *(Brethren Press, 1985), and numerous publications related to religion and aging, spiritual well-being, and other topics in the sociology of religion.*

inability to see, touch, smell, taste, or hear a phenomenon does not prove its nonexistence. Beauty, joy, happiness, grief, and sorrow are subjective or intangible, yet they are "real" to our human experience.

There is considerable nonscientific evidence that human beings are spiritual. Much of it comes out of religious and philosophical sources. The ancient Greeks separated the body from the spirit in a dualistic emphasis that made the two parts oppose each other. The ancient Hebrews, on the other hand, had an holistic emphasis that treated the soul or spirit as the essence of the person. The word *nepes,* usually translated "soul," appears 754 times and *ruah* for "spirit" 378 times in the Hebrew Bible (Old Testament). The Christian New Testament refers 146 times to the *pneuma* or "spirit" and eleven times to the *psyche* or "soul." H.D. McDonald's article on the doctrine of man in the *Evangelical Dictionary of Theology* (Baker, 1984: 676-680) adds that many other concepts (heart, mind, inner and outer nature, natural and spiritual man, etc.) also relate to the human spirit, but that there is no metaphysical dichotomy between body and spirit in the Bible. Contemporary recognition of the unity or wholeness of the human being represents, to some extent, a return to ancient wisdom. Only by analytical abstractions can we distinguish the overlapping concepts of the "spirit" and "soul" from the body and mind.

Circumstantial evidence of other kinds also lends support to the belief that the human spirit is a reality. Each person views himself or herself as an autonomous being with the ability to make decisions through an internal subjective process. Each has a certain depth of personality which illustrates that human life is much more than the sum of bodily parts. Knowing a person involves more than merely knowing about that person. Even theological proofs for the existence of God, the Eternal Spirit, have a bearing on the subject. There is a nearly universal desire among all peoples to make an ultimate commitment which theologians interpret as a longing by creatures for their Creator. The human search for meaning, self-identity, and explanations for the trials and problems of living is integrally related.

Testimonials, case studies, interviews, and questionnaire responses of those who believe in the spiritual nature of humanity constitute another type of evidence. Many religious groups have the means to test the validity of alleged relationships of the human spirit with Deity. The use of sympathetic, introspective, and intuitive understanding *(Verstehen)* in social science methodology adds valuable insights about internalized aspects of the social self which relate to the biblical concept of "spirit bearing witness with spirit" (Romans 8:16; see I Corinthians 2:11-12).

All of the evidence mustered by believers to "prove" that humans are or have "spirit" cannot convince those who choose to disbelieve. The same can be said of the alleged evidences that the "spirit" is merely a reification or mythical fantasy; sincere believers are not convinced. Two kinds of faith are battling each other. To assume that there is no God, no spiritual, and nothing supernatural is just as much a metaphysical faith as believing that there is.

This chapter accepts the historic assumption of the Judeo-Christian religion that human beings are spiritual. Along with the Italian social scientist Luigi Sturzo (*The True Life.* London: G. Bles, 1947), we view the natural realm as existing within the "atmosphere" of the supernatural in which all people live, whether they realize it or not. All are "spiritual" even if not all are "religious."

Since the spiritual encompasses the very essence of our humanity, it is difficult to define it without reducing it to something less than it really is. The spiritual certainly pertains to one's inner resources, the ultimate concern around which other values are oriented, and the central philosophy of life. It represents the totality of commitment—to God, other people, oneself, and the universe. Therefore, as the National Interfaith Coalition on Aging has expressed it, "Spiritual well-being is the affirmation of life in a relationship with God, self, community, and environment that nurtures and celebrates wholeness."

Spirituality is not merely a private internalized feeling nor a set of individualized beliefs. Likewise, it cannot be confined to the public activities in religious institutions, despite the fact that these usually are oriented around the ultimate goal of awakening and nurturing the spiritual lives of participants. Rather, spirituality flows out to all of life's relationships and concerns, merging into holistic wellness that eventuates in complete health, including security, peace, and prosperity.

Religiosity of the Aging

Sixty-eight percent of all the civilian, noninstitutionalized adults in the United States, and seventy-five percent of those past the age of fifty, claim to be members of a church or synagogue, according to a 1984 Gallup Poll. Other poll findings show that twenty-four percent of those over sixty-five pray to God three times a day or more, compared to nineteen percent of all adults. Ninety-five percent of those aged sixty-five or more who participated in a 1982 poll said they pray, and more than four-fifths claimed their religious faith was the most important influence in their lives. On a scale of zero to ten, sixty-seven percent rated themselves in the three highest categories for leading a Christian life, yet eighty-four percent wished their religious faith were stronger. Despite greater incidence of health and mobility problems, the elderly had higher rates of attendance at a church or synagogue, with forty-nine percent attending in an average week, compared to forty-one percent for all adults. Other studies have shown the elderly to be more orthodox and devout believers and to engage in personal devotions more often than younger adults.

There is no reason to believe that institutionalized older people have substantially different religious orientations, except for attendance at religious services, from those polled. Despite the general neglect of this subject in gerontological and geriatric literature, these statistics themselves indicate that a sincere concern for the total well-being of patients or clients demands giving attention to the spiritual domain of their lives. At first glance, this does not seem to be an easy task. Our pluralistic society respects religious liberty, tolerates what many call heresy, prizes individualism, and institutionalizes the separation of church and state. These barriers to spiritual effort can be turned into benefits, however, by wise action appropriately adapted to meeting spiritual needs within specific organizational and social settings.

Spiritual Needs in Late Life

Many spiritual needs are accentuated in late life. Fears and anxieties about the future easily expand from molehills into mountains of despair when one experiences physical decline and deterioration of the body, loss of friends and family members who move away or die, discrimination against the aging in social life and employment, and the increasing cost of living as inflation takes its toll. The myths of aging, which imply that the course of life in the later years is exclusively negative and downhill, may affect the elderly person's self-concept. The hour of death is ever nearer; fears of the dying process, as well as of what lies beyond the grave, may subtly infect one's equanimity. So, too, the elderly person may feel he or she is ready to die and may question why God does not allow death to occur. The fact that one has not attained goals established earlier in life may bring disappointment.

Self-concepts also are influenced by one's current circumstances and living conditions. Some have not yet resolved the questions of "Who am I?" and "What is the meaning of my life?", questions that lead directly into the issue of the meaning of the universe itself. All too many, especially when shut in at home or institutionalized for chronic disability, feel that they are useless and unwanted, a drain on society or on their families, giving nothing in return for services rendered.

The theological, liturgical, social, and psychological resources of religious faith offer spiritual help to cope with these and other needs. Without them, none can fully attain holistic well-being. When programs, agencies, and institutions that serve the aging neglect the spiritual domain, they deprive their clients of the most important source of meaningful living, dignity, and self-worth.

The Neglect of Spiritual Care

Despite the central importance of spirituality to life satisfaction and holistic well-being, it is possibly the most neglected area of care both for the frail elderly who are institutionalized or homebound and for the "young old." It is assumed that the elderly are so firmly established in their spiritual and religious (or anti-religious) orientations that intervention can bring no improvement. In fact, many caregivers assume that meeting the more tangible needs automatically results in satisfying spiritual needs as well or that the aging can find their own spiritual resources through whatever channels they individually choose.

If, in addition, administrators and staff members believe that "the spiritual nature of humanity" is merely a time-hallowed figment of the imagination or a social construction of reality, it is even more likely to be ignored. Those who lack a personal religious faith are especially prone to the conclusion that such faith is unimportant for others as well.

Educational and professional training programs generally give no explicit attention to spiritual well-being, thus compounding its neglect. Professional research reports and instructional literature related to spirituality are only gradually accumulating. Most of the materials are elusive because they are in obscure and widely scattered sources. While clerical training represents one exception to this, that training includes relatively little information on aging, and some clergy have become so strongly oriented to serving important ethical needs that they fail to nurture the human spirit.

Even agencies that attempt to satisfy the spiritual needs of clients or residents may fall short. If they assume that everyone in the agency is responsible for helping to nurture spiritual well-being, the old adage that "Everybody's business is nobody's business" sometimes proves true. If they employ a chaplain or pastoral care specialist, others may leave the entire task to that one person who, for various reasons, is unlikely to meet the spiritual needs of some. If they encourage volunteers to provide the spiritual ministries, the service is likely to be spotty and irregular, failing to serve many.

The religious and ideological pluralism of both American society and the populations served by most programs for the aging adds complexity to the problem. Although "spiritual" is not the same as "religious," there is considerable overlap in the theologies or theories, resources, and methodologies advocated for spiritual development. As a result, we are tempted to conclude that Christians are incapable of fostering the spiritual growth of Jews or Moslems, that Protestants cannot meet spiritual needs of Catholics, that the laity are excluded from spiritual ministries to which only the professional clergy are called, and that secularists can do nothing to help meet the spiritual needs of those whom they serve. Yet, within limits, every one of these generalizations is a myth that contributes to spiritual lethargy in human service agencies and institutions. With wholesome motivation and appropriate training, staff members of all religious faiths can contribute to the spiritual welfare of their patients, clients, or residents.

Research on Spirituality

Although systematic research related to spirituality is in its infancy, the bits and pieces available on the subject all point in one direction: nurturing the spiritual development and serving the spiritual needs of older people have overwhelmingly positive impacts on their lives.

Those who regularly attend religious services, as well as those who engage in private religious practices, have lower risks of mortality than those who do not. Their morbidity rates from ailments like myocardial infarction, hypertension, and smoking- or alcohol-related cancers are lower than those of people who are "less religious." Within each category of chronic illness, elderly men who say they get no strength or comfort from religion have greater functional disability than those who do.

Subjective religious experience reduces the incidence of depression, especially among men. Among women, participation in public religious activities plays an even stronger role in reducing feelings of depression. Hence, we can conclude that the higher the level of religiosity, the lower the level of depression.

Religious commitment has not only a direct impact upon wellness indicators but also indirect consequences of improving social ties with other people and providing a spiritual base for an inner sense of self-worth, a feeling of continuing purpose in life, hope for the immediate and ultimate future, and comforting mitigation of anxieties and fears.

Sociopsychological research has shown that the higher a person scores on measures of spiritual well-being, the more likely it is that he or she will score high on measures of self-esteem, perceived social competence, positive feelings about life, purpose-in-life, personal rather than ethical orientation to religious commitment, and intrinsic religiousness (as opposed to religiousness for the goal of some external or social gain). In contrast, spiritual well-being relates negatively to measures of depression, loneliness, selfishness, and individualism.

Spiritual nurture contributes to improved life satisfaction and quality of life, improved health, reduced functional disability, lower levels of depression, and thus, presumably, better general morale, smaller dosages of medications to produce the same results, and increased length of life. Although explicit cost accounting studies of comparative experimental design research have not yet been conducted, to my knowledge, these consequences suggest that it is cost-effective to provide explicit spiritual care ministries for the aging and elderly.

At the National Intra-Decade Conference on Spiritual Well-Being of the Elderly in 1977, the late Eugene R. Gonzalez-Singh reported the findings of a study of elderly mentally ill patients in a state hospital. Two groups, one

Jewish and one Roman Catholic, were involved in a therapy program that gave explicit attention to the symbols and rituals of their religious heritage. Comparison groups of other Jewish and Catholic patients had similar religious preferences, medication, and therapy but lacked the religious culture treatment. The results showed that religious therapy brought clear improvements in memory, appetite, interaction patterns, depression, and somatic complaints. The religious therapy group was hospitalized two to three months less, had more contact with reality, and had fewer somatic and depressive symptoms upon leaving the hospital.

The nursing profession has begun to recognize the importance of spiritual needs. It has incorporated "spiritual distress" into its diagnostic classification of physical and mental illnesses and disabilities. It has sponsored workshops and training programs to help nurses understand the spiritual needs of patients and develop the resources and skills to deal with them. It has initiated research projects that are demonstrating the significance of spiritual variables in coping techniques, the healing process, and wellness. The profession's experiences and findings provide insights and guidelines useful to personnel in all of the human services.

Guidelines for Spiritual Care

Probably the most important single element in serving spiritual needs is the recognition by all personnel that those needs are important. In-service training can help staff appreciate the ways in which spirituality relates positively to both programmatic and institutional goals and to the desired outcomes of their own respective specialties. It can help them to recognize symptoms of spiritual wellness and illness, to notice the indirect ways in which people give evidence of spiritual problems, and to know about feasible approaches for meeting spiritual needs through their own intervention or that of others. Training should not be limited to supervisory and professional personnel. Often the greatest amount of staff contact time, and sometimes the most emotionally intense and fulfilling association with patients or residents, is carried out by the housekeeping staff and aides who rank low in the organizational hierarchy. Because of staff turnover, it is important to include spiritual concerns in the basic orientation for newcomers, as well as to have regular reminders and refresher training.

Spiritual ministries are needed for the staff as well as for clients. When done well, they help to reduce the incidence of burnout, increase the vigor needed to perform duties well, enhance sensitivity to the needs of those who are served, and stimulate spiritual growth that results in personal benefit as well as more effective service. When employees view their work as a stewardship entrusted to them, they are more likely to have a sense of accountability and of pride in that work. This makes even menial tasks a part of their calling or ministry, not merely a routine job.

To say that spiritual needs are everybody's business is not to say that they should not have more explicit attention from certain persons. The governing board or chief administrator should appoint someone on a part- or full-time basis to serve as the director or coordinator of spiritual care. This person need not be from the ordained clergy but must have spiritual sensitivity and the ability to provide imaginative leadership. Major responsibilities can include training staff, identifying appropriate referral linkages, coordinating spiritual activity programs among residents (Bible study groups, prayer circles, self-help ventures for people with specific types of problems, hymn sings, worship services, etc.), assessing residents' spiritual growth, establishing contacts with religious agencies and community programs, and sensitizing volunteers to clients' needs and to appropriate methods of satisfying them. He or she need not personally provide these specialized services. Many can be delivered by other staff members, visiting experts, or volunteers from within or outside the agency.

Helping older people to see ways in which they themselves can help others, even if they are confined to bed or a wheelchair, may be one of the greatest services to enhance life satisfaction and spiritual well-being. The words of Jesus are especially applicable to the goal of a personal sense of fulfillment: "It is more blessed to give than to receive" (Acts 20:35). An important area of service is enabling and encouraging the vulnerable to see how the power of their listening ear, their words of encouragement and cheer, their prayers on behalf of people near and dear, and their willingness to let others serve them constitute continuing contributions to God and humanity. As they serve others, even in minuscule ways, their own self-worth is enhanced.

The coordinator of spiritual care, in consultation with the medical, nursing, and other staff members, may develop appropriate techniques for including notations about spiritual needs and therapies on the records of clients. Periodic appraisals of spirituality are just as appropriate as regular appraisals of physical and mental health. Staffing conferences should include attention to spiritual progress and regress; such attention will usually reveal significant interactions among the physiological, emotional, social, economic, and spiritual spheres of life.

The spiritual care coordinator can draw from the expanding reservoir of resources for ministering to spiritual and religious needs. In addition to the conventional tools of various religious organizations, there are:

- the literature and guidelines produced by most major denominations for ministries with the aging
- publications and audiovisual materials regularly described in NICA

Inform (published by the National Interfaith Coalition on Aging, P.O. Box 1924, Athens, GA 30603)

■ techniques like the autobiographical life history process developed by B.J. Hateley and colleagues at Andrus Gerontology Center of the University of Southern California, Los Angeles, CA 90089-0871

■ the many models for ministry developed by Dr. Albert E. Dimmock at the Center on Aging of the Presbyterian School of Christian Education, 1205 Palmyra Ave., Richmond, VA 23227

■ the resources flowing from Dr. Thomas B. Robb and other staff in the Presbyterian Office on Aging, 341 Ponce de Leon Ave., N.E., Atlanta, GA 30365

■ periodicals like the *Journal of Religion and Aging* (subscriptions: The Haworth Press, Subscription Dept., 75 Griswold St., Binghamton, NY 13904) and *Senior Update* (St. Anthony Messenger Press, 1615 Republic St., Cincinnati, OH 45210-1298)

■ services offered by the Interreligious Liaison Office of the American Association of Retired Persons, 1909 K St., N.W., Washington, DC 20049

■ the resources of gerontology centers in colleges, universities, and theological schools.

Many of the available materials were prepared primarily for local religious bodies, but they can be useful to institutional care programs and agency projects in numerous constructive ways. Linkages with congregations and other religious agencies in the surrounding community can be mutually beneficial for all who are involved. Out of them may come intergenerational ventures for children and foster grandparents, volunteer visits to residents who have no close family members, and service projects both by and for the aging.

In most communities there is need for appropriate orientation of the clergy and lay leaders of the religious congregations from which an agency's residents or clients come. Orienting these congregational representatives to the nature, goals, and services of the agency, home, or program can spread goodwill and improve the public relations image. It also can ensure that these representatives will not undermine agency goals when they visit their members and will help them to be more astute, sensitive, and constructive in their relationships with older people they contact. Not all clergy and lay leaders who attend an orientation will find that the institutional environment suits the needs of members of their congregations; however, these congregational representatives may be quick to recommend the home to elderly persons whose interests and tastes mesh with the facility's mission. Thus, even seemingly negative results of orientation and appreciation programs for community leaders can have a beneficial effect.

As is obvious from many of my comments, much more research is needed on the role of religion and the consequences of spiritual care for the well-being of residents, clients, staff, and patients. Cooperative projects with the faculty and students of neighboring colleges and universities can help fill that gap. The spiritual care coordinator may be the most appropriate agency representative for such studies.

Precautions

It is unrealistic to rely upon the rabbis, priests, and pastors of churches in the community to meet all spiritual needs of institutionalized people. Typically, their work load is already so great that they cannot take on more responsibilities without neglecting other significant tasks. In addition, the majority of clergy have not had professional training to assist them in ministering to the aging and elderly. Some may even suffer from gerontophobia, an unconscious fear of their own aging that makes them avoid association with the elderly who are chronically ill or disabled. Yet, in some instances, a pastor of a small church or an associate minister in a larger one may be the best qualified available person for paid employment as a part-time director of spiritual ministries.

If the appointment of a spiritual care coordinator is misconstrued as meaning that only he or she is responsible for all spiritual care ministries, much of the benefit may be lost and many who need spiritual care will not be served adequately. Rapport is especially important in the intimate sharing of innermost feelings and beliefs that pertain to the religious and spiritual life. One person cannot possibly establish that rapport with everyone. What that one person may not be able to do for some persons may well be accomplished by sensitized nurse's aides, cleaning persons, recreation supervisors, or fellow patients who are encouraged to reach out spiritually to others.

In all spiritual care services there must be no attempt to coerce some particular form of spirituality or style of religiousness. Spiritual growth is a product of voluntary response, not compulsory compliance. Respect for free will and the liberty to deviate from dominant religious patterns must be protected as long as they do no harm to others. However, it is well to remember that feelings of spiritual well-being are not necessarily the same as having spiritual well-being and that not all that professes to be spiritually constructive actually has the desired results. Research can help us identify erroneous approaches and harmful techniques for enhancing spiritual well-being.

Conclusion

All agencies that profess to provide total care for their residents or clients are failing to meet that goal if they do not have an explicit program of spiritual care. The methods and means they use for nurturing spiritual well-being will vary by sponsorship, clientele, goals, and settings, so no single blueprint for action will apply to all. Programs sponsored by religious organizations usually have specific beliefs or dogma, liturgies, and other commitments. These ought not to be undermined by subtle comments, nonverbal communications, or other behavior of staff members who hold contrary values.

If widely divergent philosophies, ideologies, or theologies coexist among the personnel of an institution or program, and if these are strongly held and propagated overtly or subtly, it may be particularly difficult to establish a satisfactory program for spiritual care. Even under such circumstances, however, the independence and autonomy of clients can be fostered by giving them the opportunity to pick and choose whatever spiritual resources seem best to meet their needs.

Spiritual care is ideally provided *with* the aging, not only *for* them. Many of them will be invigorated and revitalized by helping others. Their own spiritual growth and life satisfaction will be nourished by showing their love for God and people through service.

Awareness of the important role of spirituality in the package of services offered to the aging will increase. As more and more lives are changed for the better through explicit spiritual care, there will be a growing sense of elation and excitement among personnel on the staffs of agencies and institutions that serve older people. They, too, will be renewed in mind and spirit, to their own benefit and to the benefit of all whom they serve.

Chapter 3

The Environment's Role in the Total Well-Being of the Older Person

Lorraine G. Hiatt, Ph.D.

Environmental Design and Service Delivery

The purpose of this chapter is to discuss holistic design, to differentiate a well-balanced holistic environment from a more traditional one, and to offer strategies for integrating environmental design considerations into planning processes. The information presented here has implications for retirement communities, apartment residences, assisted living residences, and health care or nursing homes. Many of the points also will be applicable to older people cared for in noninstitutional residences by family caregivers.

General Definitions

Holism

Holism refers to the idea that integrated systems are more significant than the sum of their parts. Suppose one is developing a set of services, policies, and facilities. Holism would suggest that the interaction of these elements creates a powerful system of care. While this interaction has been the magic of effective continuing care retirement communities, there are implications for holism in each setting the older person occupies, whether this is a room, a building, or a full-service retirement residence.

This chapter suggests that holistic health care is offered when an environment capitalizes on the strengths or residual capabilities of older individuals and compensates for weaknesses or needs. Such care considers more than the medical needs of an individual and suggests that the experience of aging is a consequence of physical, psychological, social, and spiritual or phenomenological attributes of the person. Through holism, the caregiver and older person gain a resourceful, problem-solving approach to aging.

Environment

The term environment, as used here, refers to:

1. **Physical features:** spaces, their shape and size; lighting, acoustics, heat,

Lorraine G. Hiatt, Ph.D., is a consultant in environmental psychology and gerontology, based in New York City.

texture, and odors; color, signs, furnishings, and their location or arrangement; utensils and tools or objects, including decor

2. **Social factors:** social characteristics of people who use the setting, including the number of people; their mix of physical abilities or needs; and their perceptual, psychological, and social practices

3. **Ambiance:** overall effects of the physical and social features on individual behavior, feelings, actions, and reactions.

What Can Environmental Design Mean to Older People?

1. Environments help shape self-image. They may communicate competence or dependency. Ideally, an holistic environment would capitalize on each person's strengths while forgiving, or not placing excessive demand on, his or her weaknesses.

2. Environments can improve the quality of life, facilitating (or encumbering) any services devised. Well-planned environments optimize learning, participation, conversation, and self-care.

3. Environments for older people may become agents in the aging process. Poorly managed background noise may render the individual agitated and unable to participate or understand. Indistinguishable, undifferentiated health care units may contribute to poor motivation and disorientation, may provide insufficient subject matter for conversation, and may cause residents to withdraw.

4. Environmental design may help prevent disability. The risks of falls, scalds, or disorientation may each be mitigated by environmental design.

5. Objects and textures may stimulate thinking, elicit responsiveness, and reinforce memory. Touching is beneficial and fulfilling. As the older person loses his or her "touch partner," the objects and textures of an environment take on added importance in communicating warmth and in evoking memories.

6. Well-selected and well-managed features of the environment may reduce agitation, incontinence, wandering, or calling out. Environmental features augment the physical, psychosocial, and spiritual components of a program. A good building alone will not provide a fulfilling old age, but, proponents of holistic care might assert, physical care alone and/or psychosocial services alone are insufficient to cope with the interactive effects of aging.

Does an Holistic Approach "Really" Require Environmental Design?

Understanding that there are interactions between physical and social attributes of service delivery is essential to effective and holistic environmental design. It is difficult to achieve a well-balanced system of caring for older people without incorporating environmental design. Conversely, the best designs may remain unrealized if they are not effectively integrated with concepts of service, management practices, and corporate (or family) values.

Both housing and nursing homes developed from 1950 to 1980 have tended to be less than holistic. On the large or macroenvironmental scale, levels of care still tend to be fragmented and environments typically are static, inflexible, and difficult to shape to changing needs. Only the continuing care retirement community begins to offer a more continuous approach to the aging. On the level of microenvironmental features, such as interior design and use of equipment, both the relatively expensive continuing care retirement communities and the more modest single-level structures typically have failed to orchestrate the possibilities of functional design.

If retirement community and nursing home sponsors do not get serious about functional design, they may find their facilities on the fringes of future competition for the most-informed clients. The home building industry already has begun to incorporate functional design features into its homes. Similarly, those who are experienced in retirement housing and health care should be integrating gerontological research into design rather than dabbling in aesthetics in a few visible areas.

Why Has Environmental Design Been Overlooked?

Historically, health care has placed a heavy burden upon both the elderly and their caregivers. Like the psychologist who conducts studies of learning in a laboratory rather than in a lifelike classroom, care of older people has focused on the elderly person and his or her interaction with family, friends, and professionals. The environmental and cultural context of people has been all but overlooked. There are myriad reasons for this:

1. Environments can be neglected because the training of those in charge has not prepared them to consider the interactions between aging and environmental design. Often, there is no advocate or informed *and* vocal supporter of environmental issues. We all feel like environmental experts; by referring to our own needs, we feel we can satisfy the requirements of older people.

2. Holistic design may be overlooked because design is overly simplified. Some become concerned solely with trivial detail, such as color, without realizing that color, by itself, may have less impact on older people than do other features such as seating arrangement, acoustics, presence of textures, or appropriately selected lighting.

3. Much of the literature used as a basis for codes and design standards has come from a "disability-specific" group perspective. Until quite recently,

design standards advocated braille markings while neglecting the needs of the majority of people with minor, multiple impairments. Few design standards reflect needs of hearing-impaired older people. Groups representing those with arthritis have made a valiant attempt to advocate designs that improve manual dexterity, but only specially designed utensils, rather than larger environmental equipment, have been provided for these people. When will we hear a presentation on Alzheimer's disease or related disorders that transcends the three heuristic stages of the disease and responds to what forgetful and impaired people *can* do, *do* respond to, and *might* find comforting?

4. Codes and standards, used as a design reference, have several weaknesses:

- Many codes are not sufficiently based upon research.

- Codes often are rooted in an understanding of singular considerations (blindness or hearing, wheelchair use or manual dexterity), not in the interactive effects of minor, multiple impairments that affect older people.

- Building codes tend to focus on objects and features (grab rail presence rather than whether they can be used effectively for safe transfer in a particular bathroom design).

- The environment has been perceived as a cosmetic whose features are insignificant.

Some codes pursue one goal, such as fire safety, to the exclusion of other needs. They may even become entrenched in outmoded details of that goal—heavy door closers, wire glass, and modified open-plan social areas, in the case of fire safety—without taking an holistic view of it.

5. It is difficult and time-consuming to find and examine information on environmental design. While it is not difficult to find architects or interior designers who have worked on facilities for older people, it can be quite challenging to find those who are open and holistic in their approach and who understand how and when gerontological information can be effectively integrated into the design process.

6. Design professionals may be part of the reason holistic design has been overlooked. Characteristically, design issues have not been accorded academic prestige since there are few doctoral-level professionals in design fields. Those conducting design research sometimes have failed to disseminate findings to those who might implement them. In part, this is because long-term care is perceived as complicated and designers do not grasp the system.

In order to overcome these obstacles to holistic design, we need some high-quality thinking, innovative sponsors and regulatory and funding agencies, and effective methods of project planning and implementation. When there are more holistic models and demonstration sites, then public awareness, evaluation research, and wider-scale implementation are likely to follow.

The Goals: Options and a Balanced Environment

By balanced environment, we refer to one that is in harmony with the needs of older people. Examples would include:

- lighting that compensates for poor vision by increasing contrast and, hence, visibility
- spaces that facilitate socializing through room shape or scale (height, size, volume) and arrangement and size of furniture
- settings that elicit curiosity, imagination, control, and choice
- environmentally induced potentials for fitness and exercise consistent with one's need.

Older people are characterized by individuality. No one prototype design, level of lighting, group size, or walking distance will satisfy all older people. Holistic thinking requires that we foster variety because we want to respond to the variations in an aging population. Sponsors can fulfill the needs of older people and also family and visitors because better design solutions will appeal across the spectrum.

Limitations of "Feature Lists" in Achieving Holistic Environments

A trip through the literature (and conferences) on environmental design might lead one to a summary sheet of notes such as the one in Table 1, which lists the attributes of older people that have implications for environmental design. While each of these characteristics can change with age, environmental design may be utilized to mitigate the impact of nearly every listed item. For example, good lighting will not return sight, but it will optimize correctable or low vision; reduction of background noise will not return hearing fully, but it will facilitate understanding and reduce agitation, thereby contributing to overall comfort.

Lists, like codes, are appealing. They treat specifics and convert concepts into details. They also are deceptive.

There is a difference between applying a few design facts and achieving an holistic approach to environmental design. While the list in Table 1 may contain more details than are typically considered in designing buildings, it may not lead one to an integrated system of services, architecture, and design. One could score 100 percent on the specifics of lists such as these (or have perfect marks on a health department inspection) and fail to meet the needs of older people. For example, one may create buildings designed for wheelchair access but not for the total needs of the older person who may wheel that chair (manual dexterity, required elbow room, distinguishable turning needs). Recipes for design often do not grapple with the interactive effects of each decision upon another.

Table 1
*Attributes of Older People That Have
Implications for Environmental Design*
(See Cautions and Caveats Regarding Use of Such Material)

Vision

1. Need for more light to maximize detail or contrasts and legibility
2. Need for light directed on and appropriate to tasks
3. Glare sensitivity; need to reduce glare
4. Difficulty adjusting to shadow or dark areas
5. Need for floor to look stable and secure through appropriate selection of materials and color that distinguish floor from walls
6. Difficulty distinguishing dark shades from each other and light tones from each other when placed on similar textures, in similar light, due to yellowing of the human lens
7. Difficulty naming colors (due to yellowing of the lens), suggesting value of landmarks other than color to facilitate orientation

Hearing

1. Difficulty hearing high-pitched sounds (signals)
2. Difficulty understanding conversation in the presence of background noise, suggesting the importance of minimizing background noise

Tactile Sensitivity

1. Need for texture to be supplied by the sponsor, especially where access to possessions (or loved and natural "touch partners") is limited
2. Need for objects and surfaces that one may touch; need for tactile variety and for an environment that communicates emotions (such as warmth) through texture

Balance

1. Need for cues—such as angles and contrasts—to reinforce a sense of balance and uprightness
2. Need for floor surfaces that respond to problems in body position, including minimizing ramps or inclines

Mobility

1. Diminished mobility, suggesting a need for appropriate fitness exercise and for motivation to sustain one's residual skills
2. Need for features to optimize mobility: handrails or leaning surfaces (chair arms and blocked grabbing surfaces)

Dexterity and Agility

1. Diminished hand strength, suggesting a need for utensils and hardware, for eating and for opening windows or doors, that can minimize both wrist twisting and the need for a firm grip
2. Slower or less-accurate responses, which can be accommodated by using sensors that allow sufficient time to clear automatic door entries or elevator doors

Topics for Consideration in Designing Holistic Environments

For architecture to respond to the comprehensive needs of older people, someone needs a clear understanding of the people and of the many ways they utilize environments. Who? My experience indicates that functional design must be understood by a decision making, sponsoring group that includes board members/owners, designers (architects, engineers, and interior designers), administrators, and representatives of each subspecialty that makes up a responsible caregiving team. A project manager can be used to collect facts, locate sources, and plan, but the group must grapple with the options.

Group members can be oriented to environmental design through attendance at workshops or use of consultants, through their own reading and touring, and through experience with facilities. Such fact finding may well lead to the development of lists of characteristics and features to be considered. However, holism results from standing back from the details and thinking about the effect or concept that one is trying to create. Consider holding a retreat, guided by someone with experience, to grapple with issues that define functional characteristics of users, programs to be offered, design implications, and design opportunities. Such a retreat might deal with the following considerations.

1. How can we optimize fitness at all levels of care or in every environment (from special rooms to chairs that encourage exercise and features that motivate movement)?

2. The common wisdom espoused in some retirement communities is that people of different ability levels will not want to interact. First, how do we feel about that concept, ethically? Second, what if this were to change? Suppose that, as the median age for each ability level becomes similar, and as health care becomes more humanized, varying degrees of interaction are appealing and valuable to both the alert and the impaired or the capable and the frail. Where can people of varying capabilities interact and around what features or props?

3. Health or "wellness" is an increasingly popular concept, emphasizing preventive medicine, exercise, diet, and self-help procedures for optimizing

one's capabilities. How can each level of care take on wellness attributes? (Presume that a wellness "suite" is insufficient; we are seeking holistic, integrated approaches to program and design.) How many ways might wellness be incorporated into program and design?

4. What about designing for Alzheimer's disease and related diagnoses? Designing holistically would suggest that offering care for people with memory losses goes beyond admitting them to a "special unit" and that people at all levels of care may benefit from social and design amenities that optimize memory and facilitate way finding and independence.

5. Security has been touted as a factor in decisions to move to housing and to health care. Holistic design may incorporate security in different ways, depending upon the traditions and cultural heritage of the populace. There are no clear-cut answers, but some combination of scale, lighting, controllable sounds, textures and color, and seating design might work with appropriate staffing to create a sense of security on several emotional levels.

6. Environmental features can be part of an overall plan to reduce stress and agitation caused, in part, by crowding (social environment), background noise, inadequate responses to privacy, and excessive restraint or inactivity. There is no recipe for an appropriately stimulating environment; through active involvement of those who schedule services and design facilities, one may evolve an approach that adequately arouses, without exceeding the capabilities of, those using a space.

7. Many organizations have a religious, geographic, ethnic, or spiritual heritage. How can this heritage be expressed in design or art? How might this design or art be incorporated with the goals of a balanced environment so that it, too, is part of the whole?

8. If aging is a process characterized by individual changes, how can the environment support independence and minimize the need for relocation to higher levels of care?

There is no one set of criteria that will help managers of new construction respond to these issues. Sponsors of existing facilities may need to "read" the images or messages that their environmental design conveys and begin to plan for changes that merge contemporary thinking with previous design. Checklists are available that help assess an existing facility and its current programs and help the facility use the information to plan conceptually (see bibliography).

A test of holistic design often comes during a facility tour. If a visitor asks about fitness, exercise, or leisure activities, the tour guide should be able to show more than just the physical therapy department or a specially equipped room. Similarly, a religious home's liturgical nature should transcend weekly services or a single religious space. A continuing care home should be characterized by continuity among daily experiences, including the scale of dining, the fixtures or window operations, the dining implements, or the hair care shop.

In the past, design attention was lavished upon lobbies, a few first-floor rooms, and dining areas. What are the areas that an older person might value and use?

1. The dining room. Can one hear to converse as well as enjoy the sensory stimuli provided?

2. The bathroom. What is the ambiance of the lavatory? Of the "tub room"? I have lived in retirement centers as part of my research and heard the following:

> "The 'tub room' looks like a janitor's closet."

> "This bathroom reminds me of a car wash; I'm the car. Bath time was a special time for me at home and my bathroom was a 'touchy-feely' space."

Maybe, you reason, a texturally enriched bathroom would slow the bathing process. Or, maybe you have other ways of humanizing the intimacy of that experience. The point: find a way to dignify people who need assistance bathing, to use bath time for the paradox of stimulation and relaxation, and to provide sources of texture to that individual.

3. A place where one can read, even with failing sight. Even with limited funds, a library might be a haven of effective lighting and low vision equipment, with easy-to-view shelves designed for accessibility as well as visibility.

An individual facility's list might include other important areas of the home or other important design considerations that are derived from the corporation's mission statement, from focus groups or group discussions, from market feasibility studies, and/or from reactions of people to existing facilities and features.

Are Facilities Considering These Needs Already?

No, they are not. Site visits to over 400 U.S. and Canadian facilities showed that the average facility may be decorated (or at least have a decorated lobby), but design that is both attractive and functional is the exception. A balanced design is one that deals with:

- minor to severe levels of impairment, from vision and hearing to mobility, agility, endurance, and memory/learning skills
- the interaction of impairments; that is, the possibility that a person may have poor sight and a slow response time or may require a wheelchair and have limited ability to reach.

Implications for Sponsors

Often people design space first and then expect programs to "fit" in. It is preferable to develop together programs and design or to conceptualize the people, the programs, and then the design. The physical environment has a real appeal to older people, community members, staff, and the public at large. For one thing, it conveys an image of or information about a facility and its program. Cleanliness to the point of sterility conveys a different message than does a building that is clean and homey. In addition, a balanced model of care gives a sponsor leeway. It suggests there is no recipe for design nor for features that a particular campus must provide. Innovation, individuality, and culturally or geographically significant concepts can be integrated into design. For the sponsor concerned with questions such as "How can I appeal to families of older people?" or goals such as "The environment must appeal to relatively young staff and older residents," holistic design affords some real help.

The administrator who recognizes that glare reduction will minimize falls, maximize attention span, and in general contribute to the comfort and independence of residents may worry that the resulting dull floors will reflect poorly on the retirement home or senior center. He or she must recognize that we notice floors because our attention is not captivated by walls or because we are avoiding the pain of contemplating people, programs, or objects. Glare or shine attracts the attention of television viewers to autos, lipsticks, table tops, and dish soaps. But it does not really indicate cleanliness, nor should cleanliness be the only message to be conveyed. By providing more features worthy of public attention, the nonreflective floor (which, by the way, may be carpeted or covered with high-grade sheet vinyl and still kept clean) will not be the only attention grabber.

What else can holistic environmental design offer? Truly balanced design also will consider staff, providing areas for relaxation and parking, facilities for storage, and dignity during clocking time. All of these become important elements in design.

How to Start

1. Appoint an advocate or several technical committees to gather information and weigh alternatives. Establish a system for making decisions quickly. Technical committees typically make recommendations; the actual decision making may fall to a smaller group. However, the relationship between those evaluating and those deciding should be close.

2. Train the decision-making group and technical committee members in environmental design through workshops, reading, or planned tours. In smaller homes, this means training people from top to bottom regarding the potential of environmental design.

3. Plan before you do. In new facilities, the building should be thoroughly conceptualized prior to drawing. This means defining characteristics of users, programs, schedules, and designs. Where the team process is at its best, the

building will have a complete behavioral/architectural program describing these characteristics and detailing each room by size, configuration, design features, adjacencies, use schedules, and furnishings.

4. Use participatory planning as a means of educating people to new options, to the "model," and to your vision.

5. Develop a "critical mass" or informed base from which facilities can be planned or changes made. One lone voice will be lost in a sea of adversaries and specialists. Be wary of ready-made plans and designs, copied from other projects, that have not been amply evaluated through techniques such as an outside post-occupancy evaluation.

6. Functional design is possible. Some changes may cost more in initial product outlay but will save money in management and operation. Those that offer cost as the only reason to overlook functional design often do not want the bother that planning and integrating program and design require.

7. Ask. It will be designed. The product manufacturer has begun to recognize older consumers, who have increased buying power and discretionary income.

8. Regulatory agencies need to learn. Rather than thrust a project before them, thus putting them on the spot, treat regulators as board members or cautious, experienced colleagues in need of coaxing. Develop a process for orienting these specialists to what you have learned. Sit on the same side of the table, rather than in opposing roles, at a state conference or in a think tank when your project is not directly at stake. One of the greatest services state associations can offer their members is to convene regular design workshops that allow project managers to consider new topics and technologies and to exchange ideas with representatives of all regulatory and financial agencies involved. Such workshops should be mandatory for the regulatory agencies.

9. Invest in planning. It represents such a small investment relative to the costs of the project, of eleventh-hour changes, or of poor decisions on the whole. Many sponsors willing to spend thousands of dollars on market feasibility studies of questionable validity refuse to spend a fraction of that amount on planning.

10. Don't be afraid to get experienced people involved. Go on retreat with people who can help you understand the details of design. Off-hand decisions on furniture, products, or their arrangement will haunt you for years to come.

11. Set up a system for evaluating, looking for, comparing, and obtaining information. Other people are thinking about the same things you deliberate. If you cannot travel (or get your board or planning group on the road), find someone you trust who has seen a lot and will share it. Talk to consumer groups that look at products or organizations that collect sources. Join a service or take advantage of printed materials and computerized data sources (see appendix).

12. Have some fun. Dream. In my initial retreat sessions, I ask people to list dreams, identify the givens, and raise the questions. We take an armchair tour of what is new. We contemplate the user (who, as of this writing, tends to be eighty, not sixty, and oriented toward programs that minimize dependency on a family). We assess what we know and develop a planning process and a procedure for staking out what we do not know and what we need. The model has significance for new projects and renovations.

13. When you cannot decide, find a way to test your ideas. Nearly everything you may want to do has been tried somewhere else. Ask several people for their experiences or develop mock-ups and models. These can be very inexpensive two-dimensional floor plans made of colorful vinyl "oil cloth" and unfurled in an auditorium or they can be slightly more refined plywood, Homosote™, or fiberboard mock-ups of an apartment or room. This is not a "model apartment"; it is a method of obtaining information on spaces, sizes, and innovative configurations. Such models will help people judge space and determine whether their possessions will fit or can transfer to a bathroom configured with some new angle.

Developing a new facility or renovating an older one is a prime opportunity to integrate environmental design. However, time after time, sponsors adopt a process that guarantees that environmental design will *not* be integrated. Such processes do not lack good ideas; they lack a systematic approach or method.

The times to integrate behavorial-based data are both at the beginning and throughout the design process. This means the schedule should be drawn up jointly with whomever will be providing behavioral input. Too often, schedules are devised by architects or project managers who presume that drawings can be "jobbed out" and plans can be developed by quickly reviewing those already fashioned by a more experienced professional. Or the sponsor or architect may presume that he or she can incorporate behaviorally based information by attending a few conferences or reading some journal articles. They may, but it is unlikely that the information will be adequately incorporated. This is because writing about concepts seldom includes sufficient detail on how to integrate specific features into the whole concept. Workshops may offer details; through your planning process, these should be honed as your concept develops.

A design project typically involves a team of professionals. Do not presume that team members will be threatened by each other. It is common today for firms to form alliances. For example, in architecture, a design specialist can join with a local firm to develop working drawings or supervise site work. It also is increasingly common for good firms to work in a collegial atmosphere with behavioral scientists. The players on a design team must meet on equal ground to decide how they will relate and how they will work out the typical overlap in their skills.

Conclusion

We seem to have information on aging and on design but have yet to combine the two effectively. By making a relatively short but intense investment in planning, we may be better equipped to create not only better environments but also a more fulfilling aging.

Appendix

Sources of Catalogs and Design Information

Most catalog retailers charge a modest fee for catalogs but offer a rebate against the first order. Prior to making direct orders, check on whether the vendor offers institutional rates and/or is a member of your association purchasing group.

Ways and Means, The Capability People
28001 Citrin Drive
Romulus, MI 48174
Contains more than 1,000 products. Items for manual dexterity are especially interesting.

Comfortably Yours
52 West Hunger Avenue
Maywood, NJ 06707
Issued at regular intervals during the year with a variety of products emphasizing texture, personal convenience, and activities of daily living.

Tools for Living
400 South Dean Street
Englewood, NJ 07631
Also issued several times a year, focused on products and utensils.

Current Sources of Product Information for Vision and Hearing Impaired Persons

American Foundation for the Blind
15 West 16th Street
New York, NY 10011
Publications lists, environmental design and self-help/design resources, lending library, films, lists of low-vision services, and material on technology and on exercise.

Carroll Center for the Blind
770 Centre Street
Newton, MA 02158
See *Aids and Appliances Review* such as the issue, "Aids for the Elderly with Impaired Vision" (Summer 1984).

Self-Help for Hard of Hearing (SHHH)
P.O. Box 34889
Bethesda, MD 20817
Information and publications on products, technology, and environments that maximize independence; magazine, *SHHH*.

Source Lists of Other Products

ABLEdata
4407 8th Street, N.E.
Washington, DC 20017
Computerized and printed source lists of products by category.

LaBuda, Dennis. *The Gadget Book*. New York: Scott Foresman, 1985.
Reviews a variety of products and lists multiple sources of each.

Design Conferences

Sponsored by most national associations in aging and their state or regional affiliates.

American Association of Homes for the Aging
American Health Care Association
American College of Health Care Administrators
American Society on Aging
Gerontological Society of America
American Hospital Association
National Council on the Aging

Also contact:

American Institute of Architects
Environmental Design Research Association
State or local Cooperative Extension Services

Bibliography

Byerts, T.O., S.C. Howell, and L.A. Pastalan, eds. *Environmental Context of Aging*. New York: Garland, 1979.

Corso, J.F. "Technology Intervention for Changes in Hearing and Vision Incurred through Aging." In *Aging and Technological Advances*, edited by P.K. Robinson, J. Livingston, and J.E. Birren. New York: Plenum, 1984.

Czaja, S. *Hand Anthropometrics*. Technical Paper. Washington, D.C.: Architectural and Transportation Barriers Compliance Board, 1983.

Fozard, J. "Person-environment Relationships in Adulthood: Implications for Human Factors Engineering." *Human Factors* 23(1981):7-27.

Fozard, J. "The Time for Remembering." In *Aging in the 1980s*, edited by L. Poon. Washington, D.C.: American Psychological Association, 1980.

Fozard, J., and S.J. Popkin. "Optimizing Adult Development: Ends and Means of an Applied Psychology of Aging." *American Psychologist* 33 (1978): 975-989.

Hiatt, L.G. "Color and Care: The Selection and Use of Colors in Environments for Older People." *Nursing Homes* 30, no. 3 (1981):18-22.

Hiatt, L.G. "Designing for Vision and Hearing Impaired Older People." In *Housing for the Elderly*, edited by V. Regnier and J. Pynoos. New York: Elselvier, 1986.

Hiatt, L.G. "The Environment as a Participant in Health Care." *Journal of Long-Term Care Administration* 10, no. 1 (1982): 1-17.

Hiatt, L.G. "Frail Older People at Home." *Pride Institute Journal of Long-Term Home Health Care* 1, no. 3 (1983): 13-22.

Hiatt, L.G. "Self-administered Checklist for Planning and Priority Setting." *Nursing Homes* 30, no. 1 (1981): 33-39.

Koncelik, J.A. *Designing the Open Nursing Home*. Stroudsburg, PA: Dowden, Hutchison and Ross, 1976.

Lawton, M.P. "Introduction and Overview to Environment." *Pride Institute Journal of Long-Term Home Health Care* 4 (Spring 1985): 1-11.

Lefitt, J. "Lighting for the Elderly: An Optician's View." In *Light for Low Vision*, edited by R. Greenhalgh. Hove: Sussex, 1980.

Marsh, N. "Perpetual Changes with Age." In *Handbook of Geriatric Psychiatry*, edited by E.W. Busse and D.G. Blazer. New York: Van Nostrand, 1980.

Rodstein, M. "Accidents Among the Aged." In *Clinical Aspects of Aging*, edited by W. Riechel. Baltimore: Williams & Wilkins, 1978.

Chapter 4

The Psychodynamics of Mental Impairment in the Aged

Herbert J. Weiss, M.D.

Introduction

The problem of mental impairment in the aged forces upon us an immediate confrontation, namely, to conceptualize the pathological processes encountered. The term "mental impairment" continues to be used interchangeably with the term "chronic brain syndrome" (CBS), and the methodology of examination continues to be directed to ascertaining the classic symptoms of the syndrome. It has been increasingly apparent over the past several years that this line of pursuit places severe limitations on our efforts when other features of mental impairment (such as the wide range of behavioral disturbances and the prevalence of mood disorders like depression) are forced upon our awareness. Historically, greater attention has been paid to mental impairment based on chronic brain syndrome than to emotional disturbances. Institutions, for one, have tended to minimize these emotional or mood disturbances because these problems often did not present themselves as management problems. We tended to ignore, or failed to recognize, the nondisruptive, rather quiet, suffering in our patients.

We must recognize that terms like "mental impairment" or "chronic brain syndrome" are, at best, descriptive definitions and have limited, restricted usefulness. The primary fundamental challenge, therefore, is not merely to respond adequately to the needs of our clients, but also to construct and generate a scientific methodology derived from psychosocial investigation of the aging process itself in combination with more purely medical and neurological studies and evaluations. Such a methodology, if sufficiently inclusive, would provide a structural framework from which programmatic extensions and applications could arise in a unified, logical way.

As medical research in the biological processes of aging has continued to intensify over the past forty years, it has been perhaps only inevitable that a corresponding increase in attention would be directed toward the emotional,

Herbert J. Weiss, M.D., is director of psychiatry at Mt. Sinai Hospital in Cleveland, Ohio.

psychological aspects of the aging process also. It is a mistake to assume that this interest in things psychological emanated from medical and biological studies *per se*. On the contrary, the growth of the psychosocial interest in the aging process really stemmed from the social consequences of aging we all know so well.

The increase in the total number of aged persons in the population brought with it, as it continues to do, an increased incidence of mental disorders. These disorders initially clogged state mental hospital systems and currently continue to spill over, and perhaps clog, homes for the aged, nursing homes, and multiple social welfare agencies engaged in the problem. While it is a familiar observation that mental impairment in the aged is increasing because more people are living longer, I suggest that this increase is deceptive based on this observation alone. The greater the interest in mental impairment, the greater the incidence of mental impairment that will be found.

The automatic conclusion that the increase in mental impairment in the aged is a logical reflection of an increasing life span is worth examining for yet other reasons. This conclusion emphasizes the physical phenomena of aging and results in the familiar stereotype that aging is synonymous with deterioration and that mental disorders, or psychopathology of the aged, are always synonymous with organic deterioration. Although it is certainly true that the capacity to reestablish the automatic physiologic regulating mechanisms of the human body does progressively fail as the years proceed, one cannot separate this diminished capacity for physical adaptation from the older person's need to adapt psychologically to his or her impaired physical function or failing social resources. The moment we introduce the word adaptation into our considerations, we have begun to shift our ground away from considerations of aging as a purely biological process and to focus our interest not only on the impairment but also on the adaptive capacity that remains. This shift in focus from determining the degree of deterioration to assessing function and capacity for adaptation is clearly holistic in its basic concept as it is dynamic in expression. It was a major component of the basic challenge of mental impairment to all of us fifteen years ago and continues to be so today.

It is only when we came to appreciate the effect of several factors—the continuing expansion of our knowledge concerning the psychodynamics of aging, the growing evidence of the greater degree of ego-adaptive capacity in the older person, the increased refinement of our own diagnostic and therapeutic skills, and the potential this held for improved service to the elderly—that all of us in this field were given sufficient cause to hesitate in the course of providing protective and therapeutic services for the elderly. In the Arden House Conference on Protective Services for the Aged of 1961, a number of us indicated the danger of attempting to equate chronological age with impaired functioning. We pointed out the wide differences among older patients in appearance, skill, strength, endurance, education, occupation, intelligence, and economic and social position. We reported that the particular physical and psychological illnesses encountered in this population ran the entire gamut of social, medical, and psychiatric diseases and that these are all too often, and incorrectly, attributed to brain damage alone. We cautioned that the traditional psychiatric diagnostic categories that can be made are too often used as an indictment of an older person, especially if these categories are not measured against the assets and potentialities, the antecedent biography, the social and economic setting, the medical and surgical problems, the motives of those concerned with the care of the older person, plus many precipitating events and parameters that patients or family members cannot weigh properly by themselves. We declared that a knowledge of a patient's symptoms is not as important as information about the modifiable ability and the medical, environmental, or emotional changes required. We concluded that there are as many kinds of senescent problem as there are people with such problems.

Categories of Mental Impairment: The Dementias

Professionals in the aging field estimate that the senile form of Alzheimer's disease now ranks as the fourth or fifth most common cause of death in the United States. These are disorders of medical progress, not simply of protracted old age. One study has reported the development of dementia in one third of patients with Parkinson's disease who were followed for six years for treatment with L-dopa.[1] The authors of this study suggest that this incidence of dementia reflected a prolongation of the course of the Parkinson's disease due to treatment that allowed emergence of the dementia. It is certainly true that the longer one lives, the greater the risk of dementia. However, people live longer largely because of medical progress and the increasing excellence of total care for the aged individual.

The dementias are classically described as disorders that are manifested by the impairment of orientation, memory, intellectual function, and judgment, accompanied by lability or shallowness of affective range. This pentad of symptoms is classic for moderately advanced dementias but may be far from evident when the disorder is mild and in its early stages. Thus, symptoms may be overlooked precisely at a time when treatment might be most effective.

There is, on the other hand, considerable evidence that dementia is overdiagnosed; that is, that functional disorders are misdiagnosed as organic, especially in the elderly. In a study comparing psychiatric diagnoses given to patients over sixty-five in three different cities—Toronto, London, and New York—the authors found that organic brain disorders were diagnosed with more than fifty percent greater frequency in New York than in either Toronto or London.[2] Although variations in the population may account for some of the differences noted, it seems much more likely that elderly New York patients with affective disorders were labeled as demented, whereas in Great Britain, where the importance of recognizing functional disorders in the aged is emphasized, patients with affective disorders were more likely to be labeled correctly.

Errors of omission and commission in the diagnosis of organic brain disease arise from multiple sources. Failure to recognize the disease when it is present, even to a significant degree, probably occurs most often simply because the examining physician fails to ask significant questions. Doctors have a tendency to assume answers, and patients with dementia seldom complain of its characteristic symptoms. Early in the course of the disease the patients are most likely to complain of somatic discomforts that may point to other diagnoses. In addition, we are all familiar with the fact that patients with moderately advanced disease may conceal their dysfunction quite skillfully by using the well-preserved social skills available to them.

Diagnosing dementia when it is not present tends to arise from other sources. If the patient appears to be markedly demented and is not, then the questions asked tend to be appropriate to investigating the possibility of organic brain disease. Usually the examiner gets answers consistent with such a diagnosis. It is necessary to pay close attention to the patient's behavior, not always to the diagnostic answers, since behavior usually suggests a level of function compatible with the severity of dysfunction revealed by a mental status examination. A much more important source of error is the unwarranted reliance on ancillary diagnostic procedures, especially computerized cranial tomography or CAT scan. Dementia remains a clinical syndrome that must be established by clinical evaluation in which ancillary examination such as psychometrics and CAT scanning play significant contributing roles. However, the diagnosis must rest upon clinical study.

Etiology of Chronic Brain Syndromes

It has been assumed that most chronic dementing disorders, especially those in the elderly, are due to arteriosclerotic cerebral-vascular disease. Most patients are almost automatically assigned this diagnosis. Do the facts support the assumption that most chronic brain disease results from arteriosclerotic disorders? At present there are significant clinical and pathological data questioning this assumption and by now the evidence appears clearly to be to the contrary.

Tomlinson's study,[3] probably the finest available, clearly demonstrates that degenerative disease plays a far more important role in the genesis of dementia than does vascular disease, and this finding has been corroborated in three more recent clinical studies. Vascular disease was identified as the cause of the dementia in only eight percent of Tomlinson's patients, whereas more than fifty percent were diagnosed as having atrophy of unknown cause, almost certainly presenile or senile Alzheimer's disease, in most cases.

By now there is a significant body of evidence suggesting that accurate differentiation between vascular disease and degenerative disease can be achieved. Dementia due to cerebral-vascular disease, usually stroke, is manifested by abrupt onset, an irregular, stuttering course, and, invariably, by symptoms and signs of focal neurologic dysfunction. Slowly progressive dementia, in the absence of acute episodes and focal neurologic signs and symptoms, almost never results from cerebral-vascular disease, although psychological features cannot accurately differentiate vascular dementia from that due to degenerative processes.

The search for etiology in dementia can no longer be regarded as a luxury. Diligent investigation can uncover numerous disorders that not only require medical treatment but may also reverse abruptly under appropriate treatment. Potentially correctable disorders include depression, drug toxicity, normal pressure hydrocephalus, benign tumor, and thyroid disease. Thorough diagnostic evaluation can be expected to identify disorders with specific therapeutic implications in more than thirty percent of the patients thought to be demented.

The foregoing statements on etiology do merit some additional expansion or consideration since the familiar stereotype of "aging equals deterioration" may tend to blind our perception. Elderly patients with a rather abrupt onset of confusion, disorientation, and clouded senses may be mistakenly diagnosed as having a chronic senile dementia or as having experienced a stroke without neurological focus when, in fact, these delirium states can have three main causes: disorders of metabolism, infection and accompanying fever, and drug toxicity. These are toxic delirium states.

A large number of elderly patients, and certainly many of those in institutional settings, possess decompensating or compensated cardiovascular disease and are sustained with digitalis and diuretic drugs. Any shift in electrolyte metabolism can push some of these people over into an acute picture of confusion, memory loss, delusional thinking, and clouded senses. Delirium states also can regularly be accounted for in cases of infection and fever.

Perhaps the single most important consideration is drug toxicity. Elderly patients are excessively medicated and often come to our attention with a plastic bag filled with multiple prescriptions administered by several doctors or simply borrowed from a well-meaning neighbor. Although almost any medication may be incriminated in the development of a confused disorder, two broad classes of pharmacologic agents most often prescribed in the care of the aged should be examined: sedative drugs and psychotropic medications. The deleterious effect of the continual use of even the mildest sedative, sleep-inducing agents is well known in the field, and the dependency of the aged on

43

such nocturnal medications hardly needs further comment. The psychotropic medications, although of very great value in the treatment of behavioral disorders in the aged, nevertheless are potent agents capable of producing serious and severe mental disturbances. Of particular importance are the tricyclic antidepressants, to which the aged show a remarkable sensitivity, even to very small dosages. The continued use of antianxiety or tranquilizing medication requires the constant alertness of the caretaking staff to the side effects I have mentioned. (See Chapter 8 for a detailed discussion of pharmacological management of older patients.)

Depression

In addition to citing the high incidence of organic brain syndromes in the aged, research studies have also indicated the high frequency of depressive reactions in these populations. Depression is the most frequently encountered psychological difficulty, and it is the disturbance that is the most frequent reason for psychiatric consultation. Depression in old age seems to be an intrapsychic process, i.e., the response of the individual to an awareness of his or her losses of function, of helplessness to master these losses, and the resultant paralysis of function.

Depression in the aged is not a reflection of the conflict over aggression and accompanying guilt that is so regularly encountered in younger age groups. While one does indeed hear the familiar attitude of self-deprecation in these patients, the unconscious meaning is less likely to result in guilt as in the older person's awareness of the loss of his or her identity. This is particularly true with the older individual's growing awareness of his or her loss of mental function.

The most prominent characteristic of depressed elderly is their joylessness. They seem to find no pleasure anywhere in life. This joylessness seems to be their guarantee of care and pity from the environment, and they appear to search for it at the expense of any pleasure. Through helplessness, the depressed aged often seek protection as if the doctor, the nurse, and the caseworker were omnipotent parents. Mental outlook often seems to get better when the staff fosters or induces the conviction, perhaps really an illusion, that the patient has mastered his or her situation, has some sense of control over it, and has gained the nurse or doctor as a personal ally. This fulfillment, when it is achieved, often is accompanied by a marked increase in self-esteem with significant evidence of attendant pleasure. If we have begun our assessment of such an individual on dynamic grounds, we can readily understand why he or she responds to this kind of psychotherapy. It is as if the regressed older person, defeated by illness and social losses, has regained a sense of his or her own power and integrity, the illusion of some sense of mastery or control over these all-important caretakers in his or her new world.

Psychodynamics of Aging and the Problem of Adaptation

In the aged, it is often most difficult to separate physical disability, including organic brain changes, from the effects of prolonged and unsolved emotional conflict that may have had its historical roots in the individual's personal history and now is brought back to the surface by the changes and stresses of old age. This is a psychodynamic conception of the aging process, which is quite different from the familiar stereotype that aging is equivalent to deterioration. It is an holistic concept that embraces not only a biological change with a total personality concept but, most important, a personality concept directed toward adaptive function. It is a concept based on recognizing the unmistakable fact that relief of emotional conflict can often ease the pressure of physical symptoms that so often dominates the clinical picture of old age. This thesis forces upon us the admission that perhaps much of the apparent deterioration of aging is the deterioration of functional adaptive capacity, not of brain structure alone, and may be the result of concomitant emotional stress.

Of course, this dynamic point of view is a most seductive one, and the therapeutic promise it seems to hold may lead to an unwarranted optimism. We cannot lose sight of the fact that loss of physical reserve is an inescapable absolute, that the process of senescence is an actual organic one that regularly appears, that the constriction of function and greater vulnerability to disease in old age is not simply an expression of emotional conflict alone. Nevertheless, this dynamic philosophy, with its emphasis on adaptive capacity, does permit us to entertain a wide range of rehabilitative and therapeutic avenues affecting the care of the aged in hospitals, homes for the aged, and nursing homes, as well as in casework agencies and in broad-scale community planning.

In summary, the primary challenge confronting us is to shift our ground away from a static, structural, deterioration point of view about mental impairment in the aged to a dynamic, functional, adaptive center of interest that would enable us to prescribe and organize effective courses of treatment and intervention.

References

1. R.D. Sweet, F.H. McDowell, J.H. Fergeuson, et al., "Mental Symptoms in Parkinson's Disease during Chronic Treatment with Levodopa." *Neurology* 26 (1976): 305-310.

2. G.S. Duckworth and H. Ross, "Diagnostic Differences in Psychogeriatric Patients in Toronto, New York, and London, England." *Canadian Medical Association Journal* 112 (1975): 847-851.

3. B.E. Tomlinson, G. Blessed, and M. Roth, "Observations on the Brains of Demented Old People." *Journal of Neurological Science* 11 (1970): 205-242.

Chapter 5

Therapeutic Communities for Holistic Treatment of the Mentally Impaired Elderly

Rose Dobrof, D.S.W.

Introduction

I am one of those people whose great good fortune it was to work with and learn from psychiatrist Dr. Alvin Goldfarb. It is now more than ten years since his death, but still, I cannot write a paper about mental impairment without thinking about him and his contribution to the field of long-term care.

Alvin Goldfarb was among the first to recognize the nonprofit home for the aged as an essential component in the service network for older people. He spent much of the last decades of his life teaching the staff of such homes about mental impairment.

In the late 1950s, before Medicare, Medicaid, and the Older Americans Act, not very many self-respecting professionals went to work in nonprofit homes. But, at that time, Alvin Goldfarb already was documenting the high prevalence of mental impairment among residents and patients of these facilities. He was among the first to define not-for-profit homes as therapeutic communities in which mentally impaired older people could be helped to make maximum use of their remaining resources in a humane, supportive, and holistic environment.

He also was among the vanguard who recognized the importance of the team approach to care of the mentally impaired and who called for an investment of facility time and money in staff development and training. In both his clinical practice and his work with staff of homes for the aged, he saw, long before many others did, the need to work with the relatives of mentally impaired older people, for their own sakes and the sake of the older patient.

Finally, Alvin Goldfarb knew fully the pain that staff experience when they are forced to witness the decrements which may change once vibrant and proud older people into dependent, confused, and sometimes difficult patients. While he believed that pain is honorable and inevitable, he also felt its sharp

Rose Dobrof, D.S.W., is director of the Brookdale Center for the Aging at Hunter College in New York City.

edge could be softened if both staff and families were helped to understand the nature of mental impairment.

Caring for Mentally Impaired Elderly

Three principles which Dr. Goldfarb taught us should, I believe, inform our work with mentally impaired older people.

- First, mentally impaired older people will do better in a social and physical environment designed to maximize their remaining psychic and mental capabilities while protecting them against environmental or interpersonal demands that are beyond their capabilities to meet.
- Second, the creation of an environment that is both therapeutic and protective requires the engagement of all staff members working as a team: aides, porters, and maids as well as social workers, nurses, doctors, and occupational therapists.
- Third, care of the mentally impaired older person requires a partnership between the staff and the family of the patient.

Let us take the first principle for granted and give immediate attention to the second.

Therapeutic Community: The Team Approach

The idea of a therapeutic community or a therapeutic milieu is not new. During World War II, in both England and the United States, psychiatrists like Maxwell Jones worked to create communities in which treatment of patients was no longer the special preserve of the professional, but rather became the responsibility of all. The idea of the therapeutic community spread. It seemed an appropriate approach for a variety of treatment settings, including children's institutions, alcoholism and addiction units, veterans' hospitals, the traditional psychiatric hospital, and, finally, the home for the aged.

Role of Staff

The challenges involved in creating a therapeutic community and the intervention strategies necessary to the creation of such a milieu have been a theme of many books and articles.* The earliest writing in the field was the impetus not just for organizational changes, but also for changes in attitudes of staff toward their colleagues and toward the patients themselves. Although these early authors wrote about the creation of therapeutic communities in

*See, for example:
Alfred H. Stanton, M.D., and Morris S. Schwartz, Ph.D. *The Mental Hospital.* New York: Basic Books, 1954.
Bruno Bettelheim and Emmy Sylvester. "A Therapeutic Milieu." In *American Journal of Orthopsychiatry* XVIII (1948).
Maxwell Jones. *The Therapeutic Community.* New York: Basic Books, 1953.

other settings—mental hospitals and children's institutions, most notably—their call for changes in the traditional patterns of work among staff pertained also to homes for the aging.

Unfortunately, the necessity for these fundamental changes continues to be a major obstacle in our effective work with staff. It is difficult for all of us to give up accustomed ways of working and traditional task assignments and patterns of interdepartmental and interdisciplinary collaboration. Additionally, we know that, particularly in our units for the severely impaired, the most numerous staff must, of necessity, be at the aide level. The design and implementation of training and supervision programs for this level of staff are not an easy task. The socialization of this staff to a sense of mission about its work is difficult.

It must be acknowledged that most of these staff positions do not offer opportunity for upward mobility; moreover, the work is often difficult and the markers for success few. It is not always easy, even for the most dedicated of staff at this level, to provide care for difficult or unresponsive impaired older patients in a humane and caring way. Even the best may become impatient, angry, or discouraged. The necessity to adhere to the institutional schedule to get every bed changed, every patient dressed, and everyone fed on schedule may interfere with the kind of individualized and compassionate philosophy of care that we espouse.

Staff development is important not just because staff needs opportunities to acquire knowledge and skill. More important, our investment in staff development articulates an attitude that the staff person and his or her work are important and worthy of development. It can be quite demoralizing when staff members are told their work is important without that importance being affirmed through staff training and development activities. It may be difficult to believe that a job that takes no continuing education is really an important job.

Staff development and training is no panacea. Yet, it can help staff at the line level develop internalized norms of responsible and humane care of institutionalized patients. Similarly, the development of a team approach, as time-consuming and administratively difficult as this is, is a necessary step in the holistic design of institutional patient care programs in our units for the severely impaired.* During team meetings, which include all of the appropriate

---

*I am quite aware that there is disagreement in the professional literature about whether it is best to have separate living units for severely impaired patients or whether it is best to mix them among the total population. I am also aware that, for many homes, this issue is academic because the home itself is not large enough to have separate units. In this chapter, I am talking about team meetings on a special unit of mentally impaired patients or team meetings in a smaller home which allow all staff to sit down and talk together about the patients with whom they have a direct connection.

department personnel and staff from all echelons of the department, learning from staff seminars and workshops can be rearticulated and reinforced, theory can be translated into action, and staff work problems can be aired and solutions discovered. In short, the "total" patient can be considered in the context of his or her total environment.

The Executive's Role

The key to successful implementation of a team approach is in the hands of the administrator. The executive must believe in the creation of such an approach and must convey that belief to staff. Time must be allocated for team meetings. The meetings themselves must be structured, and there must be follow-up to guarantee that decisions reached are implemented. If the administrative sanction for a team approach is not matched by willingness to invest staff time in team meetings, and if meetings are unstructured and have no agenda and no closure, the team approach may exacerbate the tensions that frequently exist among our departments.

In emphasizing the role of the executive, I would not want to convey the notion that I believe that teamwork can be achieved through executive fiat. While the executive must be behind the effort, the team approach does not simply "appear" because the executive has "ordered" it. Team meetings at one home in which I worked took place for a year and a half before any staff below the department head level were involved. It was a long time before the team meetings really "won their spurs" in the home's system.

For example, for a long time the occupational therapist, the social workers, and the recreation professionals were likely to attend the meetings regularly, the nurses less regularly, and the doctors not at all. This said something about the home's "pecking order," but it also pointed out which departments valued a team approach in the home. It was a long time before even the nursing department was willing to protect forty-five minutes a week for the team meeting on each unit.

Conclusion

Working with the mentally impaired is a very difficult task and offers relatively few rewards and small markers of progress. The team has a unique capacity to support staff effort for the mentally impaired. I firmly believe this is essential to our work.

Staff/Family Relationships

Role of Families

Because of a long-standing commitment to holistic care of the elderly, nonprofit homes pioneered in the development of the family group before it became fashionable. Groups for families of new residents and home-wide family councils seemed to be the most prevalent types.

One project, initiated in the late 1970s by Florence Safford at the Isabella Geriatric Center in New York City, established groups for the adult children of mentally impaired older people. The program began with several assumptions:

- First, adult children have the most difficulty adjusting to their parents' aging when those parents become impaired in old age. Children can live with wheelchairs and any other kind of disability for their parents, but when mental impairment robs the children of the parents they knew, they experience a most complete agony.

- Second, the incidence of mental impairment is particularly high among people over eighty-five. The adult children of these mentally impaired patients often are beginning to face their own particular crises of old age and may be unable to cope with their own life cycle tasks and at the same time give the loving and consistent support their parents need. It should be remembered that the children of the mentally impaired elderly in non-profit homes are often in their late sixties and even their seventies.

- Third, Isabella's support group would provide a unique climate in which adult children could learn about mental impairment while using the group as an unmatchable source of mutual support.

- Finally, supporting families and helping them support impaired relatives can bring additional benefits in staff morale. It is difficult for staff to feel that only they care about the mentally impaired elderly. Staff morale can be enhanced by the symbolic value of the presence of the children, even if there is little or no communication between the old person and the children.

Conclusion

On the same grounds I argued for staff training and a team approach, I would argue for a substantial investment on the part of the home to support work with the children of the mentally impaired. In addition to the "one-on-one" contact between the nurse, doctor, or social worker and the family, a support group for the families of the mentally impaired is a particularly effective intervention strategy.

All of us who have worked with the spouses, children, and other family members of mentally impaired older people know of the pain they suffer, a pain that does not go away but lodges in their hearts and minds for as long as their impaired relative lives. These families need our help for their own sakes and they also need help to continue to support their aged relatives. And, finally, they need our help so that when their mentally impaired family member dies and their tasks are done, they have the comfort of knowing that they did all they could, and this comfort can sustain them for the rest of their days.

The investment that a home for the aged makes in staff training, in the team approach to the work, and in work with families will "pay off" in higher staff morale and a more holistically integrated program of services delivered to the mentally impaired in our homes.

Chapter 6

Innovations in Programming for Mentally Impaired Elderly

Ira C. Robbins, A.C.S.W.

Over the years, distinguished practitioners in various fields have offered thoughtful discourses on the care of the mentally impaired aged. However, none has yet to offer the "answer" to what has become long-term care's most challenging dilemma. Whatever our homes for the aging do to care for the mentally impaired must evolve from our personal philosophies and perspectives. Those perspectives are shaped not so much by the flood of information we receive as by how we choose to utilize that information. Care of the mentally impaired aging remains an art form; within the field, one can find few universally accepted truths.

Theoretical Basis for Programming

This paper originally was presented in 1978 to describe a program of care for the mentally impaired elderly at Beth Sholom Home in Richmond, Virginia, which I administered. From time to time, others have suggested that we were innovative in our philosophy and approach. If that is so, it is because we had the opportunity to learn from all the experts in the field and to design a package of programs which we could manage ourselves and which made sense to us. We did not attempt to define mental impairment; we dealt solely with what we saw.

In our collective acquisition of experiences, we were influenced by several philosophies and finally used an approach that embodied an awareness of stimulation-response mechanisms, the impact of sensory deprivation, the importance of accurate and adequate communication, the environment, and the human response forthcoming from a concerned staff. In retrospect, our approach was fundamentally holistic.

Stimulation-Response Mechanisms

When we began our program, we sought to make an impact on that multitude of aged impaired people who sat aimlessly in wheelchairs and made no at-

Ira C. Robbins, A.C.S.W., is executive director of The Montefiore Home in Cleveland Heights, Ohio.

tempt at interaction. Reality Orientation (RO), a program first used by Veterans Administration hospitals to help recovering psychotic patients grapple with the transition from institution to community, offered us a way to stimulate these patients and, we hoped, get a response.

RO, basically a mechanical procedure of repetition, is designed to reinforce time and place orientation. We expanded on this approach by replacing the role of repetition with specific stimuli that would elicit specific, active responses. For example, an orange brought into a group could stimulate conversation when patients talked about its shape, color, and use, and could titillate the senses when patients touched it and even tasted it.

Sensory Deprivation

For years, researchers have suggested that newborn infants in a stimulus-deprived environment do not do well. Stimulation is the key to development of meaningful living for human beings of all ages. This stimulus-deprivation theme played a role in our program.

Importance of Communication

Effective communication, or the lack of it, may determine what is construed as appropriate or inappropriate behavior. In a home for the aging, that communication can come through the patient's surroundings since, as Leon Pastalan wrote in his 1971 paper, "How the Elderly Negotiate Their Environment," the environment is organized like a language, punctuated with behavioral cues which can be perceived and responded to.[1]

Communication also can come from other human beings who notice us, become aware of our potential, and show an all-important concern for our well-being. Each of us has experienced the profound impact on people's lives that an untutored, unskilled volunteer can have. This simple, non-professional interaction represents an unharnessed source of help to the mentally impaired. If organized effectively, it can be used constructively.

The Environment

If "iatrogenic" refers to physician-suggested or induced disease, many of us may have created "institutrogenic" problems for mentally impaired, unwittingly inducing some of the mental impairment that we see at the institutional level.

Staff

The success of our programs for the mentally impaired, specifically the RO groups, showed us that whatever we wanted for residents, impaired or otherwise, could only be realized if we had a concerned staff. While theory would tell us that residents are an administrator's primary responsibility, I would suggest, like Rose Dobrof, that the welfare of staff heads the list of executive responsibilities. If staff members feel they have value to us as individuals, that the home is concerned for their well-being, and that the board of directors and administrator share this view, we need not be concerned about the well-being of the residents. A staff that feels cared for can reflect a caring attitude for others. Unless staff members experience a sense of self-worth, they cannot contribute to a resident's self-worth.

Programmatic Stimulus

Reality Orientation

Initially, Beth Sholom attempted to create an environmental and programmatic awareness of the needs of the mentally impaired by creating a position for a Reality Orientation coordinator. The staff person, originally hired on a twenty-hour basis (later increased to thirty hours), had two major responsibilities: the creation of RO groups and the training of RO leaders; and the implementation of a twenty-four-hour RO philosophy for all staff.

The RO coordinator was responsible for mobilizing staff to create a milieu of concern and awareness throughout the facility. Additionally, she worked to ensure that the physical environment contained enough familiar perceptual cues to minimize time and place disorientation. Residents were helped to increase their self-awareness and functional independence wherever and whenever possible.

It was important that the RO program be seen as a total staff undertaking, not merely as a nursing responsibility. To reach that end, the facility created a Think Group consisting of the administrator, assistant administrator, social worker, director of nursing, activity coordinator, in-service education director, volunteer services coordinator, and RO coordinator. The purpose of the group was to create a consensus about an institutional philosophy toward the mentally impaired and to develop program elements to be implemented and supported by all staff.

To emphasize the facility's commitment to total staff involvement, all staff were exposed to three sessions of integrated RO training. The sessions helped define the special needs of the aged and attempted, through lecture and role playing, to help staff understand the impact of sensory deficits and their relationship to communication. RO concepts—as they related to both the small groups and the total institution—also were introduced.

Attempts were made to broaden the staff base of the RO groups themselves. RO leaders, who received release time from their job responsibilities for at least one-half hour per day, five days per week, included RNs, LPNs, nursing assistants, housekeepers, dietary managers, dietary aides, executive secretaries, personal assistants, and graduate and undergraduate college students. Upon completion of the training sessions, all staff members were awarded certificates, which proved meaningful to those who previously had not been certified for anything.

Those persons ultimately selected to become RO leaders received pins identifying their leadership position and were recognized during National Nursing Home Week. The result was increased self-esteem for many staff.

Social Interaction

The RO groups were only a part of the general program for the mentally impaired. Other elements, including "Coffee Socialization" and the "Rolling and Strolling Club," were created to provide individualized stimulation beyond the structure of the formal RO groups. Without such purposefully directed opportunities for social interaction, we felt the impaired elderly would be dehumanized.

Coffee Socialization

Coffee Socialization provided an opportunity for all staff and residents to socialize for fifteen minutes per day. Between 10:00 and 10:15 every morning, all work at the facility came to a grinding halt. All staff members were expected to leave their assigned duties and report to one of our three nursing units. Coffee was available and each staff person was expected to have his or her coffee in the company of a resident, providing social interaction and stimulation. This assured at least fifteen minutes of individually programmed activity each day for a mentally impaired resident within the context of a social experience.

As with the RO group, this activity promoted self-esteem among staff. Too often, professional and administrative staff can justify elongated coffee breaks because they discuss work-related issues. Quite the opposite, elongated coffee breaks for line staff are seen as "goofing off." Line staff's participation in this work-related activity supported the notion that they have value as human beings and are capable of interacting with residents on a social level. (To clarify, this activity did not replace the line staff's coffee break but was taken in addition to that break.)

Rolling and Strolling Club

Each resident was assigned to a staff member—called the "Focus Friend" —who was responsible for wheeling or ambulating the resident within or outside the building for at least fifteen minutes per week. This one-to-one relationship gave each staff member an essential sense of personal responsibility for the humanized environment.

Physical and Mental Stimulation

In other programs at the home, we emphasized the necessity of providing high-level stimulus-provoking opportunities for residents.

Exercise Groups

Residents who were incapable of any self-directed activity without leadership took part in one-half hour of exercise every morning. Exercises were done in a seated position and were repeated daily in the same sequence, with only the music changing. Staff believed the exercise program helped residents by teaching them to identify parts of the body, increasing physical dexterity as well as tolerance and range of motion, lessening the need for sleep during the day, and, for some, increasing alertness.

Bus Rides

Residents experienced different environmental stimuli during daily bus rides that lasted from one-half hour to an hour. The rides were not an easy undertaking, but the difficulties did not seem to be disconcerting to staff. Some effort was required to put on outer garments and some residents needed to be lifted onto the bus. Some residents were unused to leaving the facility and needed to adjust to the experience of motion and the cacophony of sounds not normally heard in the home. Most patients were incontinent.

In the early stages of this program, I served as one of the bus drivers and was able to learn an important lesson about how differently each of us perceives the environment. On one occasion, one mentally impaired resident began screaming and protesting that we were going too fast. While we were probably not moving more than five miles an hour, this resident had probably not experienced motion in six years.

Animals

Animals borrowed or purchased from shelters and pet shops helped residents expose their senses of sight, touch, and smell to different stimuli. The institutional environment hosted a fawn, lamb, calf, rabbit, and the more common cat and dog. The Health Department was aware of our efforts in this area. However, we never sought its endorsement or approval and never had a prohibition applied.

Nursery School Visits

Beth Sholom opened its doors to children in the mid-1970s when we allowed a local nursery school to use our activity shop for four weeks. We reaped the benefits in terms of sensory and stimulus response, learning quickly that young children have not developed preconceived notions about the mentally impaired aged. They don't respond emotionally to debility, as others sometimes do. They are warm, affectionate, and attentive and can almost always elicit an appropriate response from the most withdrawn, impaired resident.

Sing-Alongs

Twenty to thirty residents gathered once a week with staff and volunteers to sing old songs and learn new ones. Music can stimulate some of the aged who seem to be most primitive in their responses. The rhythm moves hands, feet, bodies; the words of old songs are remembered, and the urge to dance returns. We observed two interesting side effects of this activity. Some nonimpaired residents, who normally would not visit the "infirmary" because of the impaired residents, came to the activity because of its festive nature. Second, some residents who seemed impervious to any stimuli responded to the singing by telling the off-key singers to keep quiet.

Woodworking

Mentally impaired men initially were chosen at random to participate in the woodworking program; later we were more selective in choosing participants. Achievements varied. Some participants produced detailed bookends, menorahs, etc. Others "simply" persevered in doing repetitive tasks. Such sustained activity is preferable, of course, to enforced idleness.

Sorting

Impaired residents in this program sorted objects based on color, size, or shape. Some residents were able to understand the task after verbal directions were given; others required closer attention. In the latter case, a staff person and resident initially worked almost as one, with the resident continuing the activity alone after a short time.

Sorting provides stimulation and activity, rather than idleness and consequent stimulus deprivation. Care must be exercised, however, that the objects used for sorting are not swallowed. It was our experience that most primitive, withdrawn people use the mouth for sensory stimulation in the same way that children do.

Baking

Like sorting, baking tasks initially were carried out on a repetitive basis with staff assistance. One resident broke the eggs, another resident stirred, another poured the flour from the bin into the bowl, and another sifted. The volunteer or staff member did the actual baking and all participated in the eating, which helped stimulate the taste sense.

Reminiscence Groups

Our experiences with reminiscence groups were fascinating. Even though mentally impaired residents might have been confused about time and place orientation (some did not respond to their own names), they nevertheless used the group leader as a facilitator to engage in meaningful conversations with one another about remembered past experiences. Were it not for the leader, who suggested a subject and moved the conversation along, their opportunity for spontaneous conversation would be limited. The leader developed some common experiences as a baseline for the conversation and allowed residents to interact meaningfully.

Special Activity Groups

With the help of an additional recreation specialist, we established six activity groups composed of five to six moderately to significantly impaired older residents. The activity groups met right in the nursing unit.

Tactile stimulation was facilitated by the use of foam balls which residents could touch, feel, squeeze, or put in their mouths. The multicolored balls were light enough to be thrown, rolled, pitched, tossed, passed, held, given to someone, or thrown at a target such as a box.

Similar activities facilitated name identification and eye-hand coordination. For instance, residents might be told to put multicolored scarves around their shoulders, on their heads, or on their laps. We attempted to use as much originality and creativity as possible to stimulate the residents and elicit a participatory response, whether it be a smile or a hand clasp.

Clinical Conferences

Our clinical conferences attempted to identify the resident's level of function and comprehension. We used our own Mental Status Questionnaire (MSQ), as well as observation and improvised techniques, to determine stimulus response and stimulus discrimination. We involved residents from the start and later included family members, who attended the conferences more frequently when the resident was newly admitted to the facility. After the resident had been in the home for a number of years, the family did not feel the urgency to participate if nothing dramatic was taking place in the resident's experience.

These examples represent some of the specific programmatic ways in which we attempted to respond to stimulus-deprived mentally impaired aged. To imply that all I have cited was uniformly implemented on a daily basis or was in place from moment to moment would be misleading. Changes in RO coordinators, department heads, and staff required regroupings, new beginnings with some, restarts with others. But there was a continuing philosophical thread—a feeling that permeated the home—that encouraged each employee to try to create a humanized environment for the elderly and a life-enriching experience for themselves as they accepted some responsibility for resident care.

Environmental Stimulus

To complement our programmatic efforts, we attempted to modify our environment within the context of available knowledge and limited resources. Many of the modifications were helpful, easily accomplished, and without significant cost:

1. We tried to dot the facility with perceptual cues that helped to minimize disorientation. Clocks were large and calendars were evident to reinforce a sense of time. The name of the facility was clearly identified on each nursing card and floor to reinforce a sense of place.

We must be fair to the mentally impaired when designing their environment. Any nonimpaired person living in the community, who has been away on vacation, who has not listened to the radio, not watched television, or not read the newspaper, can be confused as to the day and time. Consider, then, what happens to the resident of the home for the aging who never gets outside the building to see its name or never sees a clock or a calendar. It is no wonder residents forget where they are or what day or time it is. We are not telling them and they have no other way to find out.

2. The institutional wall provided orientation and constant stimulation wherever possible. To reinforce a sense of self, we displayed large photographs of our residents close to the areas where they resided. These displays were intended both as perceptual cues for orientation and as reinforcement of self-esteem. (Interestingly, some of our confused people inquired about their own pictures.) Other pictures were part of a museum that rotated throughout the facility.

3. We celebrated resident birthdays, sometimes individually and sometimes in groups, and made sure all residents and staff knew whose birthday occurred on any given day. Conspicuously posted signs provided staff with the necessary knowledge to communicate their greetings effectively. We also made sure residents knew when staff birthdays occurred.

Conclusion

Beth Sholom's service program for impaired residents did not have universal relevance. It reflected, instead, an attitude or philosophy by which 100 staff members developed a sense of community with 110 residents. In this community, staff responded to their own feelings of recognized worth; they provided a humanized, stimulus-enriched environment that positively affected the lives of our mentally impaired aged. We made no definable attempt to research or validate this, but we saw the value of our program in the staff's sense of purpose, in its genuine concern for residents, and in the absence of apathy and indifference.

Reference

1. L. Pastalan. "How the Elderly Negotiate Their Environment." *Environments for the Aged*. A Working Conference on Behavioral Research, Utilization, and Environmental Policy, San Juan, Puerto Rico, Dec. 17-20, 1971.

Chapter 7

The Role of the Cultural Arts in an Activities Program for Alert and Mentally Impaired Elderly

Cheryl Riskin, M.Ed.

A Tree

A tree is like a person.
It's got hands
and all its faculties.
It's got a mouth.
It stretches out its branches to enfold anyone.
A tree is like a woman.
She changes her dress often
And she's graceful.

Seashells

They're a mystery to me.
Their shapes, their sizes
They don't form any facial expressions
Or anything like that —
You have to imagine them.

This seashell is lonely,
All alone. And no one gives a damn.

Something Beautiful

My grandchildren, they're beautiful
Like pieces of china
They are great big dolls
I don't think there is anything more beautiful
Than a baby.

These poems were written by a ninety-one-year-old, mentally impaired woman at the Jewish Home for Aged in Detroit. They were created during a special project, funded by the Michigan Council for the Arts, that sought to involve nursing home residents actively in appreciation and enjoyment of the cultural arts.

Cheryl Riskin, M.Ed., is assistant director of the Jewish Home for Aged in Detroit, Michigan. When she originally shared this material in a presentation, she was the home's arts project director.

In this chapter I will discuss the importance of cultural arts programming to the elderly, including the mentally impaired, and will share some specific details regarding the arts program which I administered at the Jewish Home for Aged from 1977-1980. These details will include a theoretical background for the use of the cultural arts in an activities program that included the mentally impaired, our program's specific goals, the methods we used to implement the program, a description of the program sessions, problems we encountered, results we enjoyed, and our funding sources.

Definitions

The term "cultural arts," as used here, refers specifically to literature, dance, drama, vocal music, orchestral music, and the visual arts. Culture is the way we live. Art is a part of that culture. Art is feeling, reacting, communicating. It is a way to experience a culture. Finally, art has the potential to integrate anyone, even mentally impaired older people, holistically into a culture.

"Mentally impaired" individuals have impaired memory, judgment, and perception of time, space, and person identification. Included in the "mentally impaired" category are persons who are not oriented to their surroundings, who are confused, who may not recognize someone whom they see daily, or who may not remember a family member who has just visited. These behaviors can range from mild, to moderate, to severe levels.

Theoretical Background

Why develop a cultural arts program that includes the mentally impaired? What needs will be served?

The institutionalized aged have experienced numerous losses: they have lost jobs, home, health, mobility, even spouses and children. In the process, they have lost an important sense of identity and self-esteem.

Art may be one way to re-establish supports in old age. Through an art form, the aged person can once again become an active participant in life, learning to be productive, to contribute, and to feel success. He or she can come to an understanding that a potential for growth always exists, even in the face of increasing impairment.

Elderly persons can use artistic expression to identify their frustration and anger, their joy and happiness. They can deal with loss, restrictions, and emotions such as loneliness and isolation. They can communicate their perceptions of their current environment and remember, particularly through music associated with holidays and traditions, those satisfying parts of their former lives.

Program Goals

Based on this theoretical background, the Jewish Home for Aged identified five specific goals for its cultural arts program:

- to increase the quality of life satisfaction among residents
- to reestablish interest in those things which once brought satisfaction and pleasure
- to create new avenues for expression
- to stimulate an awareness among the mentally impaired of where they live
- to enhance socialization—among residents and between residents and staff—through involvement in an art form.

The Jewish Home for Aged envisioned a cultural arts program that would involve six artists-in-residence representing literature, dance, drama, vocal music, orchestral music, and visual arts. The program would include lectures, demonstrations, workshops, live concerts, and displays. Artists would meet residents in groups that varied in size and in levels of complexity and intensity. The groups would accommodate any individual need, interest, or ability among the residents.

Artists would be instrumental in helping residents explore different aspects of each art form, including its history, its use, society's influence on the art, and the respective techniques and methods used. Emphasis would be on discovery and experimentation and on creating an environment in which all residents would be able to experience satisfaction and interaction with others.

The program would focus on all that was still healthy and strong in the individual. It would allow each participant, regardless of any physical or mental condition, to continue to be productive, to grow, and to contribute to the art experience he or she had chosen to pursue.

Implementation

The first step in implementing the cultural arts program was the establishment of an advisory committee composed of residents, staff members, and community members who were involved in the arts. The committee suggested program content and future direction; it also recommended the names of artists who should be considered as potential artists-in-residence. The committee closely guided the program in its early stages, and individual members continued to offer comment and support after the committee stopped meeting formally.

All six artists-in-residence were practicing artists. Two had had prior experience as artists-in-residence in other settings; the remaining four had similar positions teaching either privately, at universities, or at the Jewish Community Center in Detroit. None had ever worked with institutionalized elderly.

All artists were given an orientation to the Jewish Home for Aged and attended a program on aging given by members of the administrative, resident services, and nursing staffs. As arts project director, I worked with the six artists to help schedule and carry out the program they had designed for each art area.

The program was open to all residents of the Jewish Home for Aged and its day program, whether they were alert and ambulatory or severely mentally and physically impaired. Residents were registered for sessions in various ways. Since the program was integrated into the home's resident activity department, inventories of resident interests—including, in some cases, histories of involvement in the arts—were available and aided staff in matching residents with interest groups. Often, nursing aides would suggest the names of residents they felt would enjoy a particular art activity. All staff showed enthusiasm in reminding residents of the programs and making sure they attended. In fact, information sharing from all levels of staff was frequently very helpful when it came to planning and evaluating any of the arts programs for the mentally impaired.

No one interested in attending a session was left out. If a resident required one-to-one contact, he or she would be scheduled with an artist in a small group. If a program conflicted with various therapies or doctors' clinics, meeting times were changed.

Session Descriptions

Individual cultural arts sessions gave elderly persons a chance to practice varied skills:

- Literature: Participants enjoyed poetry, creative writing, and short stories. In the poetry sessions, the artist wrote down the thoughts people expressed verbally and later read this poetry aloud. In short story sessions, the artist read a selection and then encouraged participants to respond to the ideas presented in the story.
- Theater: Each theater group involved between fifteen and twenty residents in rehearsing and performing short plays. Impaired residents learned mime and offered a special performance for all residents. Theater group participants also enjoyed performances by a local senior citizens' theater group that visited the home.
- Vocal Music: The artist-in-residence worked to help groups and individuals learn new songs and relearn songs they knew in the past. Residents experimented with rhythm instruments, learning to listen for and identify the beats in music; some accompanied our choral group. The artist also arranged for the group to listen to a number of live and recorded concerts and brought in musical instruments that residents discussed and attempted to play.

- Visual Arts: Small groups of four to five mentally impaired residents periodically received guided tours of month-long art exhibits set up in the home's main lobby. Residents also had the opportunity to meet exhibit artists during receptions held in their honor. Session participants exhibited their own work as well, painting supergraphics on pieces of masonite that were later hung throughout the facility.

- Dance: Participants in this session realized early that they did not have to be on their feet to dance. Residents often participated from wheelchairs using only their arms and hands. The artist-in-residence, on occasion, brought members of her own dance group to the facility and organized social dances in the evening. The dancers helped the mentally impaired relearn dances from the past and also taught new steps.

Periodically, all cultural arts group activities were integrated through a general theme. One year we celebrated Women's Week at the Jewish Home for Aged with an art display of works created by women. Residents listened to music composed by women and heard poetry and stories written by women.

Problems

One of our greatest problems in implementing the arts program was scheduling the artists. The daily routine of mentally impaired patients often was filled with activities with which our workshops often conflicted: resocialization classes, work activity center programs, or activities in the hobby shop. There was no way to avoid this. Finally, we identified the group of people whom we wanted to reach with each art session and scheduled sessions at times when those people would most likely be available. The artists arranged their schedules around those of the session participants.

Given the home's busy activity calendar, finding adequate locations for sessions also posed a problem. It became necessary to look at areas not commonly used for activities, such as sitting rooms or sections of lobbies.

Other problems, encountered in any activities program, included transporting groups of people to an activity or helping community members work with different home departments to set up art activities. To keep these situations from interfering with the implementation of the program, we found it best to integrate the cultural arts program into the facility's general activities program.

Program Evaluation

We developed an ongoing program evaluation process to assess such factors as resident involvement and reactions to any of the ideas, techniques, or methods that were introduced in the art sessions. We also evaluated the appropriateness of each session. Was it too long? Were new concepts introduced clearly and with an understanding of the experience level of all participants? Was each session helping to meet the overall goals established for the cultural arts program?

One year after the arts program began, I worked with the six artists-in-residence to conduct a major evaluation of the program. We found that, for our program, no one art form clearly stood out as being the best suited for the mentally impaired elderly. No one art form evoked the most response or brought about the most enjoyment or pleasure. Each art form, at some time and with some people, was successful, meeting one or more of our goals. Conversely, each art form, at some time and with some people, failed to meet program goals.

One factor was fairly consistent: residents with previous positive experience with the arts were most likely to attend an art session and to become readily involved in that session. Level of mental impairment had little bearing on how a person responded to a particular art session.

The following observations were made for each art area in which sessions were held:

- Literature: The literature groups elicited a great deal of response from almost every participant and served as a catalyst for interaction among the residents. Discussions were characterized not only by comments on the literature but also by comments on what other people in the group had said. We found the poetry sessions particularly successful with the mentally impaired, opening the lines of communication for those least able to communicate verbally.

- Theater: The theater segment was the most difficult to adapt to the skilled nursing home setting. Because of problems in memorizing parts or projecting voices, residents read their lines and held microphones. We also found the greatest need for privacy in this area, probably because we were asking a resident to participate by becoming the center of attention. Sensitive to this need, we held our sessions in an enclosed area, which eased most residents' apprehensions.

- Music: Music was the easiest way to reach the resident. Music from the past almost always elicited a response, whether it be a smile, physical movement, or actual singing along. At times it was also the stimulus for discussion of memories and feelings that the music awakened. Most residents, from alert to impaired, were receptive to hearing new kinds of music, including electronic contemporary music.

- Visual Arts: Trips to the in-house art displays and receptions with artists helped make the visual arts workshops a social experience for residents. That socializing extended to the studios in which residents created their own art and in which they displayed an eagerness to help one another.

- Dance: Dance was a special addition to the arts program. It brought together music, movement, an awareness of body parts, colorful costumes and, in some cases, a knowledge of history. It also introduced the important element of touch as staff people took residents' hands and put their arms around them to dance and draw them into the art experience. The occasional social dances organized by the artist-in-residence and members of her dance troupe helped with reminiscence, as mentally impaired residents discussed dances they had done and ballrooms in which they had danced years earlier.

Funding

In 1976, the Michigan Council for the Arts established a confined audience program as one of its top priorities for the coming year. It was the first program of its kind in the nation to bring art to people who had limited or no access to it. The council committed itself to allocating a certain portion of the money it received from the National Endowment for the Arts for the purpose of bringing meaningful, quality art experiences to confined individuals.

In 1977, the Jewish Home for Aged received a $6,000 grant to fund a six-month pilot confined audience program. The home was to match this amount on an in-kind basis, providing, in like value, staff assistance, materials, office space, equipment, and anything else necessary to carry out the program. The project, one of the first five funded by the council and the only one established by a nursing home, began in June 1977.

A second grant of $12,000 funded the program through November 1978. The home was required to match the amount with both in-kind and cash expenditures, the latter equal to one-quarter of the entire project budget.

A similar grant for $8,500 continued the program through September 1979; the fourth and final grant for $5,900 (four was the maximum allowed in this program) funded us through September 1980. Funds received for the cultural arts program totaled $32,400.

In applying for these grants from the Michigan Council for the Arts, we provided information in five major areas:

- a description of the planned arts program
- a list of community resources and organizations which would be involved with us in this program
- our reasons for developing the program
- possible future sources of funding so that the project would continue once council funding ended
- the project budget.

Those contemplating the establishment of a confined audience program should first contact their state arts council. State councils often award small and major grants, particularly when local artists are to be involved. State councils also can be a resource for information on arts organizations which have funds available for such projects. The National Center for the Arts and the Aging, whose director can be reached in care of the National Council on the Aging in Washington, D.C., is another source of information on grants for arts programs for the elderly.

Continuing the Program

When funding by the Michigan Council for the Arts ended, the Jewish Home for Aged developed several ways to maintain its cultural arts program:

- Because of the success of the original arts program, the home was given a $20,000 cultural arts endowment by a private benefactor. The endowment's interest is earmarked for arts programming.
- We obtained materials for programming which activity staff members could present when artists were not in the building. For example, the artists-in-residence in orchestral music helped us develop a library of records and filmstrips, the latter dealing with operas and operettas.
- We continue to identify artists who seek the experience of working with the elderly and can volunteer their time and talents to our residents. A volunteer continued the poetry and literature project for a few years and, last year, introduced the program into our home which opened after the formal cultural arts program ended. The Jewish Home for Aged now employs a music therapist and dance therapist.
- Our auxiliary, convinced of the benefits that residents derive from the arts, developed a fund for arts programs in the home. Designed to ensure that the arts would always be accessible to our residents, the fund has been used to finance several one-time cultural events. These include programs in dance, visual arts, and music organized by several members of the program's original advisory board.
- In a related area, the Levine Institute on Aging, the home's educational, research, and teaching arm, has recently been awarded $117,000 by the Michigan Office of Services to the Aging to provide cultural arts programs to minority nursing homes in Detroit.

I would like to conclude with a poem that was written by one of our artists-in-residence.

What I Learned From the Old People

There are some things in life
That are so precious and rare
That they cannot be handled in reality

They cannot be touched.
So fragile and good,
So delicious,
Touching would crumble them,
And make them disappear.

Such things and such beauty
Take the form of imagination.
And only in imagination can they
Remain real.

The poet, the artist, the creative person
Transcends that beauty
And gives it substance,
Very much like a person
Picking daisies from a wild field,
And gathering them into a lovely bouquet.

Chapter 8

Medication Management of Older Patients

Peter V. Rabins, M.D.

An eighty-nine-year-old woman, who was in good mental and physical health except for severe arthritis, came to an orthopedic surgeon with debilitating knee pain. Evaluation showed that replacement knee joints would diminish the discomfort and improve the patient's mobility.

The patient was followed for about one year by the orthopedic surgeon. She seemed to understand the risks of surgery, and he agreed to offer it. The surgery itself went well, and there were no anesthetic complications. However, postoperatively, the patient was confused and remained disoriented, irritable, and unable to participate in her physical rehabilitation therapy for one month.

A psychiatric consultation was obtained, and the patient's history of psychological good health was confirmed. During an examination interview, the patient was drowsy and needed to be awakened several times. She knew she was in a hospital but did not know the name of the hospital or the city. She could give no description of recent events in her life. She was unable to learn new things but could read a sentence, write, follow a three-step command, and copy a complex diagram.

A diagnosis of delirium was made. Although there were no EKG changes or other complaints of physical symptoms which are part of digitalis toxicity, the only potential physiological explanation was a dosage of digoxin (0.25 mgs per day). A digoxin level was obtained and it was markedly elevated. The dosage was diminished and the patient recovered over the next few weeks. She has been able to cooperate fully with her physical therapy program, has returned to normal cognition, and continues to do well.

This case example illustrates several issues which this chapter will discuss:

- First, even those drugs not described as "psychotropic" can have significant effects on behavior, mood, and cognition. In this case, digoxin was causing a delirium in which cognition was significantly impaired and behavior disordered.

Peter V. Rabins, M.D., is an assistant professor with the T. Rowe and Eleanor Price Teaching Service, Department of Psychiatry and Behavioral Sciences, Johns Hopkins University, Baltimore, Maryland.

- Second, proper diagnosis is the key to proper drug treatment. When a diagnosis of delirium was made, based on the patient's presentation, a careful search for a metabolic or toxic etiology could be initiated.
- Third, older persons are very sensitive to certain side effects—delirium, for example—of drugs. The changing physiology which causes this sensitivity must be taken into account in prescribing medications for the elderly. In this case, the dosage was too high for the patient's age.
- Finally, sudden changes in behavior and cognition often have identifiable physiological explanations.

General Principles of Psychotropic Drug Use in the Elderly

Indications for Medication Usage

In the broadest context, medications are prescribed for two reasons:

- A specific diagnosis has been made for which a specific pharmacological treatment is known.
- The patient is suffering certain symptoms for which drug therapy is indicated.

It is preferable to prescribe medications for the first reason. For example, a patient with fever, chest pain, and cough, who is suffering from pneumococcal pneumonia, would be treated with penicillin since this is the treatment of choice for pneumonia. Occasionally, medications to lower fever or to diminish chest pain are indicated as well. However, the specific treatment of the pneumonia will lead to cure, whereas treatment of the symptoms may well suppress the body's response to infection and even lead to death.

The treatment of symptoms also would be a mistake for the patient who complains of agitation, sleeplessness, and a general sense of feeling bad. Instead of treating the agitation with an antipsychotic drug, the physician should treat the underlying disease. This disease could be "pseudo-dementia," a form of severe depression common in older people, which affects behavior and cognition. Treatment would most likely lead to a reversal of the mood disorder and recovery. The patient can be helped by symptomatic treatment of agitation or sleeplessness while the depression is being treated. However, such symptomatic treatment should be stopped as soon as possible, with the antidepressant treatment continuing for six months to one year, if the patient responds.

Misdiagnosing the patient, or not recognizing the depression and treating only the agitation, would be a serious error since the patient might not recover and could continue to suffer the disorder even though the associated sleep difficulty and agitation might be lessened.

In truth, we often must treat symptoms. In conditions such as dementia of the Alzheimer's type, for which we have no cure, we treat symptoms when we manage behavioral disturbances with medications. In spite of these exceptions, I believe it is conceptually useful to distinguish between the two distinct reasons we use medications.

Physiologic Changes in the Elderly

Persons prescribing and administering drugs to older persons must be aware of the changes in physiology that commonly accompany aging.

Kidney function is a prime example. The ability of the kidneys to clear a given volume of blood diminishes by approximately fifty percent between ages twenty-five and seventy-five. Thus, any drug that is eliminated from the body primarily by renal excretion should be prescribed in lower doses.

Digoxin is one important example. In the case of the patient described at the beginning of this chapter, the dose of 0.25 mgs per day (the usual dose given to many young, middle-aged, and older persons) caused a toxic delirium. This was not initially recognized because the physician was not used to treating very elderly patients and did not have a high level of suspicion which the knowledge of changed renal physiology requires. Fortunately, we are able to measure the amount of digoxin in the blood stream and use this information to determine whether the dose prescribed is appropriate.

Other changes in an older person's metabolism must influence the physician's prescribing habits. Attention must be paid to the point at which specific drugs reach "steady state" levels. This usually occurs after approximately five half-lives, a half-life being the time it takes for a given dose of a drug to be fifty-percent eliminated. This calculation is very important for drugs that have long half-lives. Theoretically, it could take up to one month to achieve steady-state blood levels for a drug whose half-life is five days. Because of metabolic changes associated with aging, many drugs have longer half-lives in the elderly.

An increase in half-life can have both harmful and beneficial effects. On the negative side, a drug's toxic effects might not appear for several weeks, making the relationship between symptom and drug less than clear to the clinician. On the positive side, longer half-lives might mean that certain drugs can be given less frequently throughout the day. It might also mean that certain drugs, which produce withdrawal symptoms when their levels in the blood stream drop, might be less dangerous in older patients who tend to keep drugs in their blood streams for longer periods.

Side Effects

Elderly individuals are more likely to suffer side effects from drugs than younger people and are three times as likely to suffer side effects from psychoactive compounds. For example, drugs that cause hypotension are particularly dangerous for older persons since a lowering of blood pressure may lead to falls. Individuals started on drugs for which this is a side effect should be monitored for the symptoms of hypotension, and a high level of suspicion should be maintained. Delirium or confusion might be the only toxic effect of a drug; it might occur at doses that rarely cause delirium in the young and must be suspected when a patient's cognition and level of alertness decrease.

Many antidepressant medications, which are among the most commonly prescribed psychotropic drugs for older persons, have side effects of both confusion and hypotension, to which the elderly are more sensitive than younger persons. Another side effect of psychotropic drugs is tardive dyskinesia, an abnormal movement disorder that most often involves the muscles of the mouth, cheeks, and tongue, but also may involve the legs, arms, and trunk. Elderly women are at the highest risk for developing its symptoms, which include slow, writhing chewing movements. Early recognition of this syndrome is important since the symptoms are irreversible in 50 percent of individuals and there is, at present, no treatment.

Side effects often are shared by many drugs. Thus, patients on multiple drugs are at risk for having similar side effects caused by two or more compounds. For example, hypotension and delirium can be caused by many drugs used in the treatment of hypertension and heart disease as well as by many antidepressants and neuroleptic drugs.

The sensitivity of older persons to drug side effects should be considered when risk-benefit assessments of prescription drugs are made. A practitioner must consider choosing drugs for which harmful side effects are less likely to occur. The physician must maintain a high level of suspicion (of the drug) if he or she hears of symptoms that suggest a problem with these side effects, and should feel secure that the reasons for using a particular drug (the indications) justify the risk that it imposes. The clinician should consider whether the lowest possible dosage is being used, whether the drug can be stopped if the patient has not responded, or whether the dose can be lowered or the drug stopped after a period of time if there has been a good response.

Drug Interactions

Some drugs can either intensify or inhibit the side effects of other drugs. For example, tricyclic antidepressants will block the activities of the antihypertensive drug guanethedine. On the other hand, Dilantin (phenytoin), an anticonvulsant medication, stimulates the metabolism of antidepressant drugs. Thus, a patient who is placed on Dilantin and an antidepressant may have to take a higher dose of the former drug to achieve a therapeutic blood level. Knowledge of such interactions is needed to achieve wanted therapeutic effects and avoid unwanted side effects.

Monitoring systems, through which careful surveillance for side effects or drug interactions is carried out, are one way to improve patient care and decrease the risk of medications. Cooperation among pharmacists, nurses, and physicians, and the use of computer monitoring of medications, should continue to be explored to maximize patient care.

Principles of Prescribing

There are several other principles of drug prescription that apply to all drugs:

- Following the advice of the ancient maxim to "first do no harm," drugs should not be prescribed if they are not needed. The decision to prescribe or not to prescribe is not always a simple one, and risks and benefits must be weighed.
- When a drug is indicated, the lowest possible dose should be used.
- The least number of drugs should be prescribed to avoid so-called "polypharmacy," the use of too many drugs.
- Drugs should be prescribed at the time of day when side effects will be minimized or used in a helpful way. For example, if sedation is a side effect, it seems logical to give the drugs once at night, if possible.

Education

It is important to discuss drug treatment directly with patients and their families. Such discussion should include the reason drugs are being used, the hoped-for results, and the possible side effects. Written literature is one important way to transmit such information, particularly to individuals who are taking a number of medications and might be prone to confusion about times, doses, and amounts.

Older people undergo slight changes in memory that are most noticeable when they must recall facts previously told to them. Their ability to remember things from a written list, on the other hand, does not diminish with age. Thus, it seems plausible (although I know of no evidence to support this contention) that writing down information about medications might improve the patient's memory and understanding of them.

Some patients are cognitively unable to comprehend why they are taking medication and what are the hoped-for results. In this case, it is especially important to discuss these matters directly with the family.

Categories of Psychopharmacologic Compounds

The following brief descriptions are not meant to be used as specific guides for prescribing drugs. Further, many of the references are clinical impressions of the author rather than proven fact.

Antidepressants

Depression, sadness, or demoralization are ubiquitous feelings experienced by all individuals at some time during their lives. Antidepressant drugs should not be prescribed anytime an individual experiences such feelings. They are indicated for major depression, endogenous depression, or vital depression. These depressive states are characterized by a pervasive, persistent depressed mood, anorexia and weight loss, sleep disturbance with early morning awakening, and delusional ideas of self-blame, guilt, hopelessness, or hypochondriasis.

The tricyclic antidepressants all have similar antidepressant potency. They cause hypotension, sedation, and cardiac abnormalities in differing amounts. Amitriptyline is most likely to cause these side effects, as well as confusion, since it is the most anti-cholinergic (atropine-like) of the tricyclics. Desipramine has fewer of these side effects. Trazodone (not a tricyclic) reportedly has the fewest. Since these drugs are equally effective, the choice among them often rests on choosing the drug with the fewest side effects or the drug with desirable side effects. (For example, sedation might be desirable for an agitated person.)

Blood level monitoring of these compounds is widely available and can direct appropriate dosage schedules. One tricyclic, nortriptyline, has a so-called "therapeutic window" or blood level range in which it seems to be most effective. When the blood level exceeds this range, the likelihood of a good response diminishes while the chances of toxicity increase. This is not true of other tricyclic drugs for which there seems to be a direct relationship between blood level and response rates until toxicity is reached. Thus, nortriptyline should be considered when the clinician is concerned about side effects and can obtain blood levels. The drug dosage can then be adjusted to maintain a therapeutic blood level for several weeks. If there is no improvement at that dosage, the drug should be stopped, since the patient probably has had an adequate trial.

Antipsychotic or Neuroleptic Compounds

These compounds were developed to treat schizophrenia and the manic phase of manic-depressive illness but also have other indications. Among the elderly they are frequently used for control of agitation, particularly in the demented individual.

Side effects are significant. In addition to tardive dyskinesia, discussed above, some common side effects are hypotension, sedation, and extra-pyramidal symptoms such as Parkinsonism, akathesia (a state of motor restlessness), and dystonic reactions (prolonged contraction of specific muscle groups most commonly of the neck, tongue, or trunk).

Antipsychotic and neuroleptic compounds can be grouped together according to their side effects; such grouping can shape clinical decisions for prescribing them. The drugs that cause hypotension are also the most sedative and cause the fewest extra-pyramidal symptoms; drugs that cause the most extra-pyramidal symptoms cause the least sedation and hypotension. As with antidepressants, the clinician often chooses a neuroleptic by its side effects. He might choose a drug for its sedating properties or because it is less likely to cause hypotension.

The extra-pyramidal side effects listed above can be diminished or abolished through the use of anticholinergic drugs such as benztropin or trihexphenadyl. The use of these drugs by persons suffering the uncomfortable side effects of neuroleptic drugs is important to improve compliance, decrease patient discomfort, and decrease the likelihood of secondary complications such as falls. However, the anticholinergic drugs also have undesirable side effects, including atropine psychosis and delirium. Patients taking these drugs must be observed carefully for increasing forgetfulness.

Antianxiety Drugs

Anxiety and restlessness are common complaints of older people, especially when they are depressed. The benzodiazepine drugs can be very useful in relieving these discomforting symptoms. However, they, too, have undesirable side effects that must be carefully monitored:

1. They sometimes cause paradoxical worsening of agitation. This side effect makes the patient more uncomfortable. But, more important, the decision to increase drug dosage when patients become more agitated might lead to further worsening of the agitation. My experience has shown this to be particularly true of the cognitively impaired or brain injured individual. Therefore, I rarely prescribe benzodiazepines for patients suffering from dementia with agitation.

2. Antianxiety drugs can have very long half-lives in elderly persons and may cause forgetfulness and delirium. Thus, the development of these symptoms one month after a drug has been started does not exclude the drug from being the causal agent.

Lithium

Lithium is primarily used to treat patients who have suffered at least one manic episode and are felt to have bipolar or manic-depressive affective disorder and antidepressant activity. Elderly persons often require lower doses and lower blood levels of lithium for effective and safe treatment. While a blood level of 0.8 to 1.2 meq/dl is desirable for younger individuals, older persons seem to have fewer side effects and often respond well at blood levels between 0.5 and 0.8. Additionally, since lithium is excreted through the kidneys, lower levels are less likely to have toxic effects.

Cognition-Improving Medications

At present, no drugs have been shown specifically to improve thinking. Vasodilators, stimulants, and vitamins all have been studied without success. One ergot derivative, dihydroergotamine (Hydergine), has been shown to improve behavior in individuals suffering from dementia. However, it does not improve memory. Research is now being conducted on a new class of compounds called nootropics, which might increase brain metabolism and thus improve cognition.

Alzheimer's disease, the most common cause of irreversible dementia, has been shown to be associated with a decrease in brain acetylcholine (or, more specifically, choline acetyltransferase, the enzyme needed to make it). Many recent studies have focused on means of increasing the amount of acetylcholine in the brain. This might be accomplished by giving drugs that are used to make acetylcholine (such as lecithin or choline), by giving drugs that decrease the breakdown of acetylcholine and thus increase the time it might act, or by using compounds that directly mimic the action of acetylcholine. While results have been disappointing thus far, definitive studies have not been conducted.

Prescribing for Symptoms

Restlessness and sleeplessness can be symptomatic of many disorders. After a proper diagnosis has been made (or occasionally before), the physician can decide whether symptomatic treatment is necessary. I believe non-pharmacologic treatment, if available, should be tried first. However, I use chloral hydrate for patients with dementia who have severe sleep disorders that endanger them and are distressing to their caregivers. If agitation is a problem during the daytime and evening, neuroleptic drugs can be used. The principles of prescribing mentioned earlier (use the lowest dose, stop if possible, and so on) apply to their use.

Conclusion

Prescribing and administering medications for older people requires a knowledge of specific aspects of the physiology of aging and a recognition of the importance of an holistic approach to the care and diagnosis of the older patient. Like most things in medicine, drugs can be of great help when used appropriately but have the potential to cause problems. Overdependence, misuse, and underuse can diminish our ability to help patients.

Chapter 9

Dental Health's Role in Enhancing the Elderly's Well-Being

Terry F. Crawford, D.D.S.

Characteristics Affecting Geriatric Dental Care

Oral health care is one of the most neglected areas of care throughout life. Only 56 percent of the population made one or more visits to the dentist in 1978. The figure was only 35 percent for people over sixty.

The major barriers to dental care among the elderly are the attitudes of the patient, the attitudes of the practitioner, physical accessibility to the office, and the financial limitations of the patient.[1]

Patient Attitudes

The elderly today can be placed in two basic groups: those born around 1900 and those born around 1920.[2] Elderly born around 1900 are more concerned about general medical health than about dental health. While the younger elderly place greater importance on dental care and preventive information, they also show a lack of concern about dental health. The attitudes of the geriatric patient run the gamut from "the old should expect aches and pains" to "losing teeth is normal with growing old." A recent study conducted in New York revealed that several groups of elderly did not consider dental care enough of a priority to place it on a list of health desires and concerns. When dental care was added to the list, it was found to be a very low priority.[3]

Practitioner Attitudes

In the past, a dental practitioner generally would "grow old with his practice," maturing along with his elderly patients. But, given recent increases in the number of elderly, this matching is no longer always possible. Unfortunately, the aged patient is something of a threat to the younger practitioner who is poorly educated in the areas of acute and chronic medical disorders that often affect the dental treatment of geriatric patients. Within the last few years, dental school curricula have been modified to include training in the treatment of

Terry F. Crawford, D.D.S., is chief of dental services at Wesley Woods Health Center in Atlanta, Georgia.

these geriatric patients. Hopefully, such knowledge will allow the young practitioner to treat the elderly patient with sensitivity and expertise.

Physical Accessibility

Making sure that the elderly person seeking dental care can physically get to the office is a major challenge for the practitioner. Buildings in which dental offices are located are not always readily accessible to wheelchairs. Only the newer dental offices feature corridors and examining areas wide enough to allow the passage of wheelchairs and walkers. If the older person is institutionalized, he or she may experience the additional hardship of finding transportation to the dental office, unless family, friends, or public transportation are available. The use of specialized transportation, such as an ambulance, can create a financial hardship.

Finances

For geriatric patients living on a fixed income, dental treatment is an "out of pocket" expense and, as such, becomes an elective treatment with a very low priority. Medicare offers minimal coverage of only some surgical procedures. Private insurance coverage to this population group is lower than that of the general population.[4]

Sociophysical Health Concerns

Dentistry and oral care, one of the least sought after areas of treatment, may be one of the most important areas of concern for the aging individual. This is because of the effect of dental health on both self-image and the overall health of the individual.

Self-Image

A person's self-image often is affected by his or her appearance, speech, and general emotional well-being and affects how the individual relates to himself and to society. It is difficult to interact and to participate in groups when one feels inadequate or less than pleasing in appearance because of unattractive teeth and poor oral health. It is difficult to smile—in a photograph or among friends—if one has missing or broken teeth. It is difficult to communicate with others when the oral structure that makes speech possible—the tongue, cheeks, lips, teeth, and palate—is impaired, causing the person to emit different sounds than the majority of the population. This difference, in fact, may lead the person to avoid or retreat from other members of society.

Physical Health

A myriad of activities and functions take place within the oral cavity. The first step in the digestive process takes place in the oral cavity. Oral fluids mix with food to moisten it, which helps in chewing and swallowing and stimulates the taste buds, creating a pleasurable experience for the individual.

Through the oral cavity we take in nutrients and expel air in the production of sounds. We use the muscles around the oral cavity for facial expressions. Its tissues experience the normal aging patterns and the pathological processes that impair functions. Since the oral cavity is located near the majority of the nervous tissue of the body, any disorder in the area can cause the whole body to be distressed or disoriented. Let us consider some of those disorders.

1. The temporomandibular joint, which allows the mouth's opening and closing, experiences great "wear and tear" over the life of a patient. Due to long-term stresses and imbalances, the joint may become a problem area in the aging individual. Incorrect occlusion of the teeth, the abrasion of the chewing surfaces due to wear, and loss of teeth will greatly affect this joint.

2. Periodontal disease of the gums is a chronic disorder that has been estimated to affect ninety percent of the population.[5] Unless recognized and treated, this disease can lead to tooth loss.

3. Dental decay or caries is still a problem for the elderly, even though it is not a major cause of tooth loss.

4. Oral carcinomas are responsible for 3 to 5 percent of all human cancer[6] and occur increasingly with age. They are most often seen on the tongue and the floor of the mouth. Carcinomas found in the oral cavity can be either the primary site of the carcinoma or a metastatic lesion from a primary site elsewhere in the body.

Function and Aging of the Oral Structures

Several structures in the oral cavity—the lips, cheeks, tongue, floor of the mouth, hard palate, soft palate, salivary glands, and teeth—are important to total human health.

Lips

In early life, the lips serve a very important role by allowing the newborn baby to gain nourishment through nursing. Throughout life, lips are important in phonation and speech as well as in the appearance and socialization of the individual.

The lips are exposed to many changes in weather over a lifetime which affect their condition. With continued exposure to the sun, the upper lip is particularly vulnerable to precancerous changes that could result in the formation of basal cell carcinoma.

The edentulous or toothless patient experiences a loss of vertical dimension in the lips. The corners of the mouth will droop and a condition known as angular cheilitis will form there. These moist areas at the corners of the mouth may also become infected with a fungus called Candida albicans. Both conditions can cause discomfort and irritability in the elderly and may affect nutrition if these areas are tender while eating.

Cheeks or Buccal Mucosa

The cheeks or buccal mucosa make it possible to maintain food on the chewing surface of the tooth during mastication. The underlying muscles are important in speech as well as in facial expression. The mucosa, while very fragile, must withstand many insults such as temperature, chemical, and abrasive changes. They can reflect changes in the systems of the body such as vitamin deficiencies and can become quite irritated when aphthous ulcers or canker sores cause extreme pain and hinder eating and speaking. The cheeks are also the sites of several other problems caused by lichen planus, Candida albicans, or trauma.

Tongue

For the infant, the tongue is critical in nursing and in the development of the taste sensation. Later in the development of the individual, the tongue plays a role in speech.

The aging tongue is subjected to many changes that affect oral and general health. Its appearance can alert the practitioner to vitamin deficiencies, and it can be the site of many ulcerations, including oral carcinoma, most often found on its lateral border. The tongue must be cleaned daily since the papillae on its surface can trap food, causing bad breath and inflammation of the papillae. Changes in the taste sensations and a decrease in the number of taste buds in the tongue mean that the elderly require larger amounts of certain seasonings — including sugar — to stimulate them. That increase in sugar accumulation can exaggerate the tooth decay process.

Floor of the Mouth

The floor of the mouth is located totally under the tongue and is surrounded by the mandible or lower jaw. The floor is important in speaking and mastication since a series of muscles used in opening the jaw lie under the floor's mucosa or mucous membrane. The ducts to the submandibular salivary glands are located on either side of the floor's midline. Their flow is important in moistening food as well as in moistening the mucosal tissue.

Reduced salivary output in the aging will cause the mucous membrane to be somewhat drier and more fragile, thereby increasing the incidence of ulceration and pain. This dryness can be exacerbated by mouth breathing due to nasal difficulty. Overextension of a dental prosthesis into the floor of the mouth also can cause great discomfort. This overextension can be caused by improper determination of the denture-bearing area or changes in that area due either to alveolar tissue shrinkage when teeth are lost or to prolonged use of an ill-fitting denture.

Palate

The palate separates the nasal cavity from the oral cavity and aids phonation and mastication. The palate consists of two parts:

- The hard palate, a thick fibrous tissue covering bone, is used as a roof of the oral cavity against which the tongue mashes the food. The hard palate is subjected to temperature, chemical, and abrasive changes and can be a frequent site of trauma. This trauma can be quite irritating, especially as the tongue moves forward each time the patient swallows.
- The soft palate, located about two-thirds to three-fourths of the way back in the roof of the mouth, prevents food from flowing into the nasopharynx. The soft palate area can become quite irritated when the removable denture prosthesis is overextended. If impinged upon, this area may be a site where a "gag" reflex initiates.

Periodontium

The supporting structure of the teeth, called the periodontium, consists of the alveolar bone, periodontal membrane, and gingival tissues. The periodontal membrane acts as a cushion between the teeth and the bone. An inflamed periodontium presents a serious health problem to the individual. Depending on the degree of inflammation and bone loss, a patient can lose good teeth due to poor support. Periodontal disease often is asymptomatic, with mobility of teeth being the first sign that the disease is present. In acute cases, a periodontal abscess may occur when calculus and debris in the mouth are forced into a deep crevice around the tooth.

Teeth

The teeth are used in phonation and mastication. While decay attacks the teeth throughout life, they become increasingly abraded and worn with age. Elderly patients are particulary vulnerable to root decay, which results from exposure of the root's outer covering (softer cementum) to the oral environment. This occurs when the gingival tissue recedes and exposes this area to bacterial attack. The tooth loss common in old age can create bite problems that affect the health of the temporomandibular joint. Failure to have lost teeth replaced can cause nutritional deficiencies and ultimately a loss of a sense of well-being.

Systemic Considerations in Oral Health

Several general health problems can manifest themselves in the mouth. These include vitamin deficiencies, diabetes, arthritis, Parkinson's disorder, Paget's disease, squamous carcinoma, and venereal diseases.

As mentioned earlier, the oral cavity may also be a primary site for carcinoma which then can spread to other parts of the body. The medical treatment of these disorders, as well as those of cardiovascular and other systemic problems, will affect the management of the geriatric individual by the dental practitioner. Therefore, the dental practitioner working in a health care facility must be holistically oriented and have a basic knowledge of the disorders that characteristically affect the elderly and must work closely with the medical practitioner and the nursing staff when treating these patients.

Geriatric Dental Care Programs

There are several important reasons for making dental care available to the institutionalized geriatric patient:

1. There is no other health professional who knows more or is better educated about the oral cavity than the dental practitioner, a professional trained both as a diagnostician and a surgeon. He or she functions as a critical member of the interdisciplinary team responsible for the total health management of the geriatric patient.

2. Elderly persons no longer take for granted that they will lose all their teeth during the aging process. A recent survey conducted at a skilled nursing care facility in Atlanta found a 6 percent decrease in the number of toothless patients in six years, due to better dental care of those geriatric patients surveyed.[7] Increased retention of natural teeth carries an awesome responsibility for directors of geriatric care facilities, who must ensure that aging individuals receive proper oral care daily.

In establishing a dental program in a geriatric care facility, attention must be paid to staff development, patient education, assessment of patient needs, determination of the facility's commitment to the program, policy development, and staff appointments.

Staff Development

Increased sweet consumption coupled with a soft diet can increase the retention of plaque, a bacterial film that covers teeth. If the individual is unable to remove this plaque due to physical, medical, or psychological impairment, decay and periodontal disease can result. Persons over forty primarily lose their teeth due to periodontal disease.

If patients in a geriatric care facility are unable, physically or mentally, to render proper daily oral health care to themselves, the effort must fall upon staff. While this may be an inordinate task to lay upon an already over-burdened work force, oral care programs have been successful when staff are aware of the importance of plaque removal and brushing and the relationship of oral health to general well-being. Staff development seminars, in which staff perform these procedures first on themselves, can be useful.

The unit manager—in most cases, the registered nurse—should be trained in plaque removal and should lead a team of LPNs and nurses' aides who will perform this task for patients. The RN also should be able to perform a cursory oral examination of his or her patients to identify abnormal situations that require the practitioner's attention.

Patient Education

The geriatric facility should have a trained team of individuals who offer information and training on oral hygiene to nonimpaired residents and to staff members required to perform oral care for impaired residents. Such education can be accomplished with the aid of dental and dental hygiene students or individuals recommended by the local dental society. In addition, several brochures that explain brushing and flossing procedures are available from the American Dental Association.

For the physically impaired, devices that alter the normal toothbrush should be employed. Clay or a tennis ball can be used to build up the handle of the toothbrush, aiding the arthritic patient who may not be able to close his or her hand tightly enough to hold a small toothbrush handle. Floss holders that require only one hand to operate can work very well in the hand of the physically impaired patient. Small interproximal brushes can be used by the staff or patients.

Oral Health Screening

Before establishing a formal dental program, the dental needs of the patient population should be determined so the level of care to be rendered can be ascertained. This can be done through the oral health screening, during which the dental practitioner uses tongue blades and flashlights to look cursorily at the condition of the soft and hard tissues.

Determination of the Level of Commitment of the Facility to the Patient

Once resident dental needs are established, the extent of the facility's commitment to dental care must be determined. Appropriate persons within the institution must decide whether a staff advisory dentist or dental board will be appointed and how extensive the dental program will be. Dental treatment programs can constitute several phases, including the initial examination, comprehensive dental care with a recall dental component, and emergency dental care.

Policy Development

Decisions must be made regarding how communications with a patient's family or guardian will be handled, what policies will be developed in the area of patients' rights, and what procedures will govern admission to the dental program.

Patients' rights are one of the most important entities in the development of a dental health policy. Patients must not feel threatened by the dental program and should understand that they will not be required to have dental treatments they do not wish to have. Communication with the family should be conducted on a person-to-person level, if possible, with pamphlets and other written material used as a backup to explain the need for routine dental care and the dental program's admission procedures.

Staff Appointments

The dental practitioner is the institution's primary agent in dental care. He or she serves as a consultant, a resource individual, and a clinical practitioner. His or her responsibilities consist of organizing and presenting programs for educational development of the staff, selecting members for and acting as a resource individual to the institution's dental health team, and delivering dental care.

Dental Services Available to the Geriatric Patient

Initial Oral Examination

The initial exam is perhaps the most important part of the services available to the geriatric patient. Ideally, each resident should be examined as a routine matter upon admission to the facility. Examination results will become part of the resident's medical file and should be related to the patient or the family for their consideration and future treatment.

The initial oral examination is important to the patient because it often comes after years of degeneration, generally due to a lack of concern. The exam should consist of radiographs and any other necessary tests, a thorough oral exam, and a review of the patient's medical and pharmacological history. Once this information is gathered, the practitioner can formulate a treatment sequence for the patient.

Comprehensive Dental Care

A treatment sequence should consist of the orderly listing of treatment priorities with the most serious conditions treated first. Once this treatment is completed, the patient should be monitored periodically and should have routine cleaning (prophylaxis) and examinations. This recall program allows the practitioner to make early observations of any changes in dental health and to work with the individual, staff, and family in maintaining that health.

Emergency Dental Care
Emergency dental care should be available to any patient in the facility. The registered nurse can evaluate the potential emergency and refer the patient to the dental practitioner, who will determine whether emergency care is needed and who will provide that care. Emergency care usually involves treating a hemorrhage, an acute infection, or a trauma to the oral cavity. An acute toothache also can qualify for emergency dental treatment since the patient's discomfort can disrupt other residents and staff.

Dental Equipment
In order to provide comprehensive dental care to institutionalized elderly, the dental practitioner must have ready access to a fully-equipped on-site dental area. This necessity may change in the future, however, as portable dental units become more widely available.

There are several ways to acquire dental equipment. The easiest and most expensive way is to order it through a dental supply house. Supply house personnel are quite knowledgeable about equipping and designing dental facilities and can offer valuable assistance in this area.

Dental equipment also can be acquired through donation of equipment or funds to purchase equipment.

The basic dental facility should include a specialized dental unit, light, and chair; a radiographic unit and facilities to develop radiographs; an air compressor and vacuum pump; and dental instruments and supplies. Consultation with a dental advisory board or a supply house can help the facility draw up a more comprehensive list.

Future Need for Dental Care
As more people grow older and maintain better dental health, and as we develop a greater appreciation for an holistic approach to health care of the aging, there will be an increased need for dental services to the elderly. As middle-aged and younger people progress to old age, they will retain more of their natural teeth and they will have practiced better home oral hygiene procedures. The ever-increasing elderly population will test health professionals and require them to increase the quality and quantity of dental care they provide. Facilities for the aging must be willing to accept the challenge and take steps to improve the quality of life of aging individuals by improving their oral care.

Notes

1. H.A. Kiyak, "Psychosocial Factors in the Dental Needs of the Elderly." *Special Care in Dentistry* (Jan.-Feb. 1981): 22-30.

2. Ronald L. Ettinger and James D. Beck, "The New Elderly: What Can the Dental Profession Expect." *Special Care in Dentistry* (Mar.-Apr. 1982): 62-69.

3. R.D. Marinelli et al. "Perception of the Dental Needs by the Well Elderly." *Special Care in Dentistry* (July-Aug. 1982): 161-164.

4. Z.S. Blau, "Socioeconomic Variations in the Dental Status in Behavior of Today's Elderly." *Special Care in Dentistry* (Nov.-Dec. 1982): 244-247.

5. H.C. Gift, "The Elderly Population." *Journal of the American Society of Geriatric Dentistry* (Spring 1978): 9, 17-21.

6. Theodore E. Bolden, "Epidemiology of Oral Cancer." *A Textbook of Preventive Dentistry*, ed. Caldwell and Stallard. (Saunders Publishing Co., 1977): 81-101.

7. Terry F. Crawford, unpublished survey conducted at Wesley Woods Health Center, Atlanta, Ga., Sept. 1982.